EXERCISES FOR
HEART HEALTH

EXERCISES FOR
HEART HEALTH

William Smith

Foreword by
Dr. Fred M. Aueron, MD, FACC, FSCAI

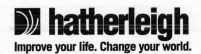
hatherleigh
Improve your life. Change your world.

EXERCISES FOR HEART HEALTH

Text copyright ©2009 Hatherleigh Press, Ltd.

Hatherleigh Press is committed to preserving and protecting the natural resources of the Earth. Environmentally responsible and sustainable practices are embraced within the company's mission statement.

www.hatherleighpress.com

This book was edited, designed, and photographed in the village of Hobart, New York. Hobart is a community that has embraced books and publishing as a component of its livelihood. There are several unique bookstores in the village. For more information, please visit www.hobartbookvillage.com.

Library of Congress Cataloging-in-Publication Data

Smith, William, 1976-
Exercises for heart health: the complete plan for heart attack, heart surgery, and cardiovascular disease recovery and prevention / William Smith ; foreword by Fred Aueron.
p. cm.
  Includes bibliographical references.

ISBN 978-1-57826-303-5 (pbk. : alk. paper) 1. Heart--Diseases--Exercise therapy. I. Title.
RC684.E9S65 2009
616.1'20642--dc22
2009018303

Exercises for Heart Health is available for bulk purchase, special promotions, and premiums. For information on reselling and special purchase opportunities, call 1-800-528-2550 and ask for the Special Sales Manager.

Cover Design by Heather Daugherty
Photography by Catarina Astrom

10 9 8 7 6 5 4 3 2 1

DISCLAIMER

Consult your physician before beginning any exercise program. The author and publisher of this book and workout disclaim any liability, personal or professional, resulting from the misapplication of any of the training procedures described in this publication.

DEDICATION

To Dr. Fred Aueron, for his professional and personal guidance. Dr. Aueron's dedication to the field of cardiology and patient care has provided me with countless examples on how to deliver the best in preventative health services and, more importantly, how to do so with the human touch.

To Dr. Gil Hedley, my mentor for countless 'inner body explorations' who taught me to think outside the standard model of the human form and view the body as one interconnected unit of continuity and function. From Dr. Hedley's teachings, and our work in the lab, the systems of the body—particularly the heart—has taken on an entirely new presentation. I consider our work together to be truly life altering as it has provided me with an all-encompassing approach to my clients' bodies, allowing me to help them improve their inner bodies while also working on their outer body through exercise.

To my clients. Wow! I don't even know where to start. You've taught me patience, dedication, commitment, and perseverance. Our time together has been a learning experience that I will carry throughout the rest of my life.

To Angela, the love of my life. You are truly an angel on earth that has been sent to watch over me as my life partner. My heart is yours, every resting heart beat.

Table of Contents

FOREWORD

Heart disease is a growing, ever-present illness in western civilization. In the United State alone, over 80 million Americans suffer from cardiovascular diseases, including heart attack, stroke, hypertension, and vascular disease. In 2004, coronary artery disease caused 1 of every 5 deaths in the United States. Nearly 2,400 Americans die of cardiovascular disease each day—an average of 1 death every 37 seconds. Nearly one third of these deaths occur in people who are 65 years old or younger.

As a practicing Interventional Cardiologist, I have spent the past 35 years recognizing the prevalence of heart disease, and reacting to its long-term effects. While much improvement has been made in treatments such as coronary bypass surgery, balloon angioplasty and coronary stents, we must still wonder why it is that the United States is still has the highest incidence of heart disease.

Although modern medicine has made significant inroads in conquering risk factors, most studies suggest that an active lifestyle is necessary in lowering overall risk. The combination of diet, proper nutrition, physical exercise and aerobic training contribute to a healthier body, longevity, and a more functional lifestyle.

In 1965, President Lyndon B. Johnson, recognizing the value of exercise and diet to the American population, started the President's Council on Physical Fitness. Reconstituted in the 1980's by Ronald Reagan, this visionary council certified the role of physical activity and diet as a national mandate for health and longevity. In 2007, the American Heart Association published Guidelines for Physical Activity and Public Health in Older Adults: Recommendation by the American College of Sports Medicine and the American Heart Association (*Circulation*, 116:1094-1105, 2007). As a guideline, this document advocates a combination of aerobic activity, muscle-strengthening activity, flexibility activity, and balance exercises in the elderly population. A plan must be established that addresses each type of activity, and care should be taken to identify how, when, and where each activity should be performed.

The great value of this book, authored by my colleague, and good friend, Will Smith, is to structure the value of your exercise program as you grow into the golden years. Exercise is not an option. It is a requirement for continued health, mobility, and function. The exercises provided in this book reflect the value of flexibility, aerobic capacity, and functional movement. They are critical to maintaining function, and are easy to do without costly equipment. You will gain a great deal of insight from reading the suggestions in these pages. This invaluable information will allow you to be more functional as you seek your fountain of youth.

—*Fred M. Aueron, MD, FACC, FSCAI*

INTRODUCTION

Can Exercise Really Help Heart Disease?

Let me open our Heart Healthy discussion with some practical advice from a gentleman who remains my role model to this day, my grandfather Bill. He offered me simple words of advice that he has used over the course of his lifetime, and wisdom which I apply to my own lifestyle as follows:

1. **Everything in moderation**
2. **Move your body every day**
3. **Feel connected to your surroundings and community**
4. **Practice portion control and be sure to get enough good fats, fruits, vegetables, whole grains, fiber, protein, and water**
5. **Stay in touch with your primary care provider**
6. **Read up on health and medical topics—become your own best resource**

These wise words have contributed to a long and fulfilling life for my grandfather. I would also note he has 27 grandkids and 8 children at the time of publication! This keeps him engaged in the day-to-day lives of his family, giving him an extremely effective motivation to keep his heart healthy.

Exercises for Heart Health is a simple system that I have developed for you to use in your everyday life. My system has been applied through years of work with patients, clients, and training sessions, and seems to work with every client I have worked with, and I am positive it will work for you too!

CHAPTER ONE

Getting to the Heart of It:

About the Causes of Heart Disease

Cardiovascular disease, an umbrella term for a variety of heart and circulatory conditions, is often referred to as a chronic illness or "the silent killer." You've likely listened to health professionals refer to heart disease as cardiovascular disease (CVD), coronary artery disease, and vascular disease, all of which are fancy terms that fall under similar heart-related diagnoses. In the 2008 World Health Statistics, the World Health Organization found that chronic conditions such as heart disease and stroke become primary contributors to increased morbidity (illness) and mortality worldwide. According to the American Heart Association in 2002, "CVD claims the lives of nearly half of the 2.4 million Americans who die each year—almost as many lives as the next seven leading causes of death combined (IDEA 2003)."

A leader in the study of CVD, Ties Boerma, commented on this recent global shift. "In more and more countries, the chief causes of deaths are non-communicable disease including heart disease and stroke, rather than the traditional communicable diseases (WHO, 2008)." Generally heart disease has been associated with affluent, industrialized societies. However, this is no longer the case as less healthy nutritional habits and decreased physical activity are becoming more prevalent across the globe.

> **"The Chronic Disease Pandemic has arrived. The World Health Organization estimates that chronic disease claimed 35 million lives in 2005. Worldwide, cardiovascular disease is the leading cause of death, followed by cancer."**
> —Michael J. Klag, MD, MPH, Johns Hopkins

The Centers for Disease Control and Prevention (CDC) lists heart disease as the number 1 killer in the U.S., with the rest of the world falling into similar patterns of mortality rates. Cancer, stroke, respiratory diseases, accidents, diabetes, and Alzheimer's complete the top of the list. As mentioned earlier, we are looking at a global shift from communicable (such as malaria and TB) to non-communicable (cardiac, stroke, neural-degenerative diseases), largely preventable diseases worldwide. As noted previously, lifestyle, globalization and various social determinants play into this equation (visit *www.cdc.gov/nchs/fastats/lcod.htm* for more information).

Anatomy of the Heart

The basic function of the heart is to supply oxygen to the body. The heart is a muscular organ about the size of your fist, and consists of four chambers, valves, and walls that separate the respective chambers.

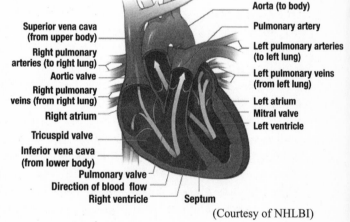

Superior vena cava (from upper body)
Right pulmonary arteries (to right lung)
Aortic valve
Right pulmonary veins (from right lung)
Right atrium
Tricuspid valve
Inferior vena cava (from lower body)
Pulmonary valve
Direction of blood flow
Right ventricle
Septum
Aorta (to body)
Pulmonary artery
Left pulmonary arteries (to left lung)
Left pulmonary veins (from left lung)
Left atrium
Mitral valve
Left ventricle

(Courtesy of NHLBI)

With each beat, the heart receives, circulates, and delivers blood from the body and lungs. Located in the chest cavity, the heart has multiple branches that bring oxygenated and de-oxygenated blood to and from the heart and then pushes this blood to the necessary organs or to the lungs.

Gil Hedley, PhD on the Function of the Heart

"The whole heart, braided with itself, the nervous tissue, and all the cells of the body, is the internal motion of life of a body. A happy heart will freely and fully refresh the vital movements of the blood, which will support all of the joyful/healthful processes of the body (gross motor/digestive/reproductive/growth). A contracted/held/depressive heart will less aptly fulfill those roles, and will lack the healthful feedback from those activities which enhance and facilitate its motions. So the state of the heart reflects the whole, and supports the whole, in feedback loops which either enhance or diminish the overall vital capacity/life expression of the person..."
—Gil Hedley, PhD, Educator

The heart is one big bundle of nerves and muscle. Just like any other muscle in the body, the heart uses a nerve signal to create contractions. This electrical signal starts in the upper right corner at 220 beats per minute (hence the number for figuring out maximum heart rate, which you can find on page 39). As this electrical signal transmits throughout the heart muscle, it reaches the bottom left corner of the heart (also known as the left ventricle), giving us a resting beats per minute rate of 60. Coronary arteries wrap around the heart, supplying a continuous blood flow used exclusively by the heart for its own needs. In order for the heart to function properly, these coronary arteries must continuously clear plaque buildup. Coronary artery disease and coronary bypass grafts are common outcomes from chronic stress on the heart.

Heart disease has many names, including cardiovascular disease, an all encompassing term that covers the heart, lungs, and vascular system. The vascular or circulatory system includes the arteries, veins, capillaries, and peripheral vessels that carry blood, nutrients, and fluid to every part of the human body. The heart is the pumping center or "centrifuge" as termed by my mentor Gil Hedley, that provides the home base for oxygenated blood returning from the lungs and deoxygenated blood returning from the circulatory system.

Controllable risk factors (such as smoking, nutrition, and inactivity) as well as non-controllable risk factors (such as family history and age) can impact the development of a condition called atherosclerosis. Atherosclerosis is defined by the American Heart Lung and Blood Institute as follows:

Does Gender Effect Heart Disease?

Heart disease does not turn a blind eye when it comes to men and women. Both genders are impacted by cardiovascular disease to varying degrees. One way to understand your gender-specific risk profile is to take a Reynolds Risk Score. The Reynolds Risk Score originated from the famous Framingham Heart Study conducted over decades in Massachusetts. Framingham's risk model used factors such as age, sex, total cholesterol, HDL cholesterol, smoking status, and systolic blood pressure. Harvard University later developed the Reynolds measurement based on an individual's level of C-reactive protein and whether the person's parent had a heart attack before age 60 (Harvard Health Publications). There are now 8 criteria for the updated Reynolds Score. Visit *www.reynoldsriskscore.org* to take your Reynolds Score.

Quick Facts: Women

Provided by the American Heart Association

- Cardiovascular disease's mortality rate in highest amongst women. Of the five diseases with the highest mortality rates, cardiovascular disease kills more women than the next four diseases combined.
- Currently 1 in 3 female deaths result from cardiovascular disease, while 1 in 30 deaths result from breast cancer.
- One in 8 women aged 45 to 64 has heart disease. One in 4 women over the age of 65 has heart disease. Currently, 7.2 million women have heart disease.

Quick Facts: Men

Provided by the Mayo Clinic

- The average American man lives 5.3 fewer years than the average woman.
- Men suffer from heart disease 10 to 15 years earlier than women do, and they're more likely to die of it in the prime of life. About one-fourth of all heart disease-related deaths occur in men ages 35 to 65.

"Atherosclerosis (ath-er-o-skler-O-sis) is a disease in which plaque (plak) builds up on the insides of your arteries. Arteries are blood vessels that carry oxygen-rich blood away from your heart to other parts of your body."

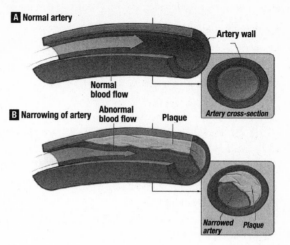

(Courtesy of NHLBI)

Plaque is made up of fat, cholesterol, calcium, and other substances found in the blood. Over time, plaque hardens and narrows your arteries, reducing the flow of oxygen-rich blood to your organs and other parts of your body. This can lead to serious problems, including heart attack, stroke, or even death.

Once atherosclerosis begins to develop, aggressive intervention is necessary for treating this disease. A proactive approach includes aggressively modifying risk factors such as smoking and obesity, undergoing a medical baseline review with your medical practitioner, and exploring the possibility of cardio-protective drug intervention.

The above diagram shows the difference between a normal artery and one with arterial plaque build-up. You can see how the opening within the vessel circumference decreases significantly as plaque build-up increases, which can negatively impact one's blood pressure and ultimately increases workload on the heart to pump blood through smaller openings.

Metabolic Syndrome and Cardiovascular (CVD) Risk

Metabolic Syndrome is an umbrella term for contributing risk factors of cardiovascular disease, and specifically the development of coronary artery disease.

As described by Dr. Richard Fargos, M.D., "Metabolic syndrome is a grouping of cardiac risk factors that include insulin resistance, obesity (especially abdominal obesity), high blood pressure, abnormalities in blood clotting, elevated LDL cholesterol and triglycerides, and reduced HDL cholesterol. Each of these factors increases the risk of heart disease, and when they are seen together, the risk becomes even higher."

Smoking (the single most common cause of preventable death worldwide, according to the World Health Organization), belly fat (measurable with a special test), hypertension, and high resting blood sugar are examples

NHLBI/AHA's Components of Metabolic Syndrome

The National Heart, Lung, and Blood Institute, along with the American Heart Association, developed the following outline of the primary contributors to metabolic syndrome.

Six components of the metabolic syndrome that relate to CVD:
1. **Abdominal obesity:** Waist Circumference/Belly Fat
2. **Atherogenic dyslipidemia:** High Triglycerides and low HDLs
3. **Elevated blood pressure:** Hypertension
4. **Insulin resistance and/or glucose intolerance:** Creates elevated blood sugar levels
5. **Proinflammatory state:** C-reactive protein (CRP) markers are high. Marks levels of inflammation, which experts now say may be the most important predictor of heart trouble. The American College of Sports Medicine (ACSM) notes persons with high CRP levels are twice as likely as those with high cholesterol to die from heart attacks and strokes. Below is a chart highlights levels to be aware of in your blood work:
>3 mg/L=High Risk
>1-2.99 mg/L=Moderate Risk
<1 mg/L=Low Risk

6. **Prothrombotic state:** Fibrinogen, a clotting agent in the blood, is found in high levels. Too much of this blood protein, which is essential for clotting, can increase your chances of having a stroke.

Three Categories of Controllable Lifestyle Contributors' to CVD include:
1. **Underlying CVD Risk Factors:** abdominal/belly fat, physical inactivity, fatty diet
2. **Major CVD Risk Factors:** smoking, hypertension, high LDL
3. **Emerging CVD Risk Factors:** pro-Inflammatory state (high CRP test), glucose intolerance

of metabolic syndrome factors. Regardless of whether you believe in classifications or categorizations, one of my basic goals is that reading this book will help you to understand the contributing factors to cardiovascular disease and how you can reduce your risk.

Since the bulk of metabolic syndrome risk factors can be altered through education and lifestyle modification, you are on the path to better heart health by reading this book. I am going to teach you how to address these metabolic and lifestyle risks so you can improve your cardiovascular health!

Coronary Artery Disease (CAD)

Coronary artery disease (CAD) is a precursor to developing atherosclerosis, a hardening of the arterial or vascular walls. This hardening leads to increases in blood pressure, resting heart rate, and an enlarging of the heart due to increased workload.

The Cleveland Clinic is a world renowned heart center in Cleveland, Ohio. According to the clinic, "Coronary artery disease is the narrowing or blockage of the coronary arteries caused by atherosclerosis. Atherosclerosis (sometimes called 'hardening' or 'clogging' of the arteries) is the buildup of cholesterol and fatty deposits (called plaque) on the inner walls of the arteries that restrict blood flow to the heart. Without adequate blood, the heart becomes starved of oxygen and the vital nutrients it needs to work properly. This can cause chest pain called angina. When one or more of the coronary arteries are completely blocked, a heart attack (injury to the heart muscle) may occur."

Risk Factors of Developing Coronary Artery Disease (CAD)

When you get a splinter in your finger, you sense pain. Unfortunately, when your coronary arteries become clogged with plaque, the first signs of discomfort could be angina (pain) or heart attack, which is why CAD is often called the "silent killer." Because CAD can come about so quickly and without warning, it is extremely important for those at risk for developing CAD to be screened and to then take steps to prevent further development of the disease.

Framingham started as a way to gather data on heart disease and stroke with the hope that by identifying the origins of cardiovascular disease. New treatment and diagnostic protocols could be developed. This has happened. I highly recommend that readers of Exercises for Heart Health visit the Framingham homepage (*www.framinghamheartstudy.org*) to view this ground breaking research.

Risk Factors for Developing CAD

Provided by the American Heart Association

Major risk factors that can't be changed:

• Increasing age
• Male sex (gender)
• Heredity (including race)

Major risk factors you can modify, treat or control:

• Tobacco smoke
• High blood cholesterol
• High blood pressure
• Physical inactivity
• Obesity and overweight
• Diabetes mellitus
• Stress
• Too much alcohol

   In this chapter, you have heard a lot about risk factors and prevention of cardiovascular disease. The following chapters will teach you how to develop a winning heart health strategy through prevention, exercise, and leisure activities.

CHAPTER TWO

Breakthroughs in Heart Health:

What the New Studies Say

An Aging Society

As America's Baby Boomer population continues to retire in mass numbers, there is an increasing need for health programs that can address this population that will undoubtedly live longer, and hopefully healthier. To better understand the impact that this population will have on our healthcare system, the federal government has awarded research grants to institutions such as the Johns Hopkins Bloomberg School of Public Health, which is leading a new national survey of older Americans and patterns of disability and aging.

"Our aim is to provide scientific evidence that can help in reducing disability and improving the daily lives of older people," said Judy Kasper, Ph.D., principal investigator of the study and professor in the Bloomberg School's Department of Health Policy and Management. "We will assemble a rich database of information that will allow researchers to study how people's ability to function independently changes over time, as well as examine the factors that influence those changes, such as social environment and medical care."

"The trend in declining disability among older Americans is an important indicator that shows that we can improve health and independence as we age," said Richard Suzman, Ph.D., director of the Division of Behavioral and Social Research at the National Institutes of Health. "We hope that this study will play a critical role in maintaining or accelerating this trend as we address the challenges of our aging population."

U.S. Healthcare System

Doctors have become increasingly efficient at keeping patients alive for longer periods of time, particularly following acute events such as heart attacks. Pharmaceuticals, post-operative care, and physical therapy have increased life spans to levels that were never thought to be possible 100 or even 50 years ago. The National Center for Health Statistics estimates the current average life span to be 78 years of age.

The U.S. Healthcare System is generally respected around the globe for having the top practitioners across various specialties while setting the pace at many of our advanced research institutions. Unfortunately, delivering this high quality care in a convenient and cost effective manner has been the sore spot currently under scrutiny by economists, patient rights activists, and governmental regulatory bodies.

The U.S. spends an estimated $300 billion each year in post-heart attack care—an enormous financial and clinical strain on our healthcare system. The good news is that heart attacks and chronic illnesses such as cardiovascular disease (CVD) can, in many ways, be prevented with simple lifestyle changes. While there are some risk factors (such as age, family history, and medical history) that cannot be changed, many risk factors including smoking, inactivity, waist circumference, nutritional intake (particularly fats and sugars), and sleep are under your control.

Utilizing the *Exercises for Heart Health* program, you can take control of your heart health by modifying these risk factors.

Longevity Medicine and Health

Heart healthy medicine has become a really big deal. As explained earlier, our population's Baby Boomers are now retiring in increasing numbers and are the largest and wealthiest generation to ever retire. Moreover, this generation wants top-quality services to keep them moving and functioning at a high level. Quality of life is paramount— without health, this affluent population segment will not be able to fully enjoy the riches they accumulated from working hard during their professional lives. This population shift has consequently increased the need for identifying risk factors and classifying those individuals who are at risk for acute or chronic cardiovascular disease.

The proposition of living longer and living better is highlighted by a quote from Dr. James Fries featured in the *New England Journal of Medicine*. Dr. Fries says, "The adult vigor can be extended well into the ninth decade of life, with illness and disability compressed into a period that shortly precedes death."

The study of living longer and healthier, also known as "anti-aging medicine" or "longevity research," is one of the hottest topics in the health care system. One very important point to discuss is the difference between longevity research/medical practices and preventative health/fitness-based longevity. While longevity research deals with areas such as supplementation, hormones, and genetic marker testing, preventative health and fitness-based approaches—like this book—offer overall recommendations to enhance your quality of life and reduce your risk factors of developing a particular disease or condition.

CHAPTER THREE

The Keys to Long-Term Heart Health

How to Keep Your Heart Strong and Healthy

Disease Prevention vs. Disease Management

Disease prevention addresses cardiovascular risk factors proactively, while disease management consists of reacting to, and treating, symptoms. Dr. Mark Hyman, a pioneer of functional medicine and an active supporter of patient-centered medicine, emphasizes the need to recognize an approach to medicine and healing that focuses on "identifying and addressing the root causes of chronic health challenges as opposed to merely treating symptoms" *(Experience Magazine, 2008)*.

Disease prevention tools such as this book help to address the chronic and debilitating impact of CVD by enabling you to assess the recognizable signs, symptoms, and risk factors and ultimately lessen the need for surgery, drugs, and clinical therapy. *Exercises for Heart Health* aims to address the root causes of chronic disease through education and application of proven fitness programs.

Respected research-oriented organizations such as the American Heart Association, American Association of Cardiovascular and Pulmonary

13

Rehabilitation, and American College of Cardiology have taken extensive steps to define what heart healthy fitness programs should consist of. The American Heart Association and the American Association of Cardiovascular and Pulmonary Rehabilitation recognize that all cardiac rehabilitation programs should contain specific core components that help to reduce cardiovascular risk, foster healthy behaviors and compliance to these behaviors, reduce disability, and promote an active lifestyle for patients with cardiovascular disease.

Risk Factors

CVD and CAD risk factors can generally be characterized as controllable or non-controllable, as mentioned in previous sections. Controllable risk factors include smoking, obesity, and inactivity. Non-controllable factors include age, gender, and family history. The overview below covers several of the most important risk factors that you should take into consideration when making your "Heart Healthy" exercise, lifestyle, and medical decisions.

Smoking

Smoking is the most dangerous risk factor. Your lungs soak up the tar and carcinogenic particles, which are then deposited into the soft tissues— including the large lung bodies. The lungs are a soft expandable organ that inflates and deflates similar to a balloon. Your lungs are responsible for converting deoxygenated blood for use throughout the body via the heart's pumping mechanism. Once your lungs are polluted with chemicals, the capacity to oxygenate blood is significantly decreased. Over time, smokers become at greater risk of developing diseases such as Chronic Obstructive Pulmonary Disease (COPD), bronchitis, and emphysema. In addition, obvious congestive symptoms, including hacking, wheezing, and jaundice can develop (U.S. Surgeon General). The lungs and heart sit next to each other, so any dysfunction in the lungs will have a negative impact on the heart (and vice versa). For example, if the lungs become polluted from smoking, their ability to achieve maximum expansion decreases, causing the heart to enlarge from a congestive build-up of inefficiency in the lungs. This leads to conditions such as congestive heart failure and fluid on the heart, essentially choking the heart muscle.

Hypertension (High Blood Pressure)

In a recent study, researchers from the National Heart, Lung and Blood Institute point out that more Americans than ever are being treated for high blood pressure. A normal blood pressure for healthy people should be around 120/80. For every 20 point increase in systolic (top number, 120 in the example) and 10 point increase in diastolic blood pressure (bottom number, 80 in the example), your risk for developing coronary heart disease roughly doubles (Shah, Princeton Medical Center)."

Another study, published by the New England Journal of Medicine (NEJM), assessed populations with risk of cardiovascular disease in persons with high-normal blood pressure (systolic pressure of 130 to 139 mm Hg, diastolic pressure of 85 to 89 mm Hg, or both).

The study concluded that high-normal blood pressure placed an individual at risk for developing cardiovascular disease, and raised the question of whether lowering high-normal blood pressure would reduce the risk of developing cardiovascular disease (NEJM, October 2001).

An increasing amount of research is also being done on the connection between race and one's susceptibility to high blood pressure. Minorities have been shown to be at greater risk for a variety of heart-related conditions, one of which is hypertension. Dr. Kevin Fiscella, M.D. released a study in 2008 that explored the various aspects of race and high blood pressure.

"Disparity in the control of blood pressure is one of the most important, if not the most important, contributor to racial disparity in cardiovascular mortality, and probably overall mortality," said Dr. Fiscella. He continues, "If we as clinicians are going to reduce cardiovascular and stroke-related deaths...we need to pay attention to all the barriers to improving blood pressure control, particularly for minority patients."

Controlling blood pressure through regular check-ups with your physician and monitoring your blood pressure through journaling will help you track your health and ultimately reach a better understanding of what you can do to prevent heart-related conditions. Movement therapies including qigong and meditation have also been shown to have a very positive impact on controlling high blood pressure. Visit the National Center for Complementary and Alternative Medicine (NCCAM) at *www.nccam.nih.gov* to learn more about these therapeutic movement approaches.

Diabetes

As more and more Americans are diagnosed with diabetes and are being placed on higher cost medications, the national cost of this disease has nearly doubled from $6.7 billion in 2001 to $12.5 billion in 2007 (Archives of Internal Medicine October 2008). This growing population of diabetics are not only at risk of various diabetes-related health problems, but are also at higher risk of developing cardiovascular disease (CVD). In fact, it is estimated that approximately 65 percent of diabetics die from CVD.

Dr. Caleb Alexander, M.D., the lead author of the Archives of Internal Medicine study, estimates that in the U.S. alone there are over 19 million cases of diagnosed diabetics. The presumably frightening addendum to this is the number of at-risk or pre-diabetics that do not control their risk factors and ultimately develop the disease.

In October 2008, the Centers for Disease Control and Prevention released new data that points to a 90 percent rise in Type 2 diabetes in the last 10 years. Known otherwise as the lifestyle diabetes, this form of diabetes is caused by lifestyle factors, such as obesity and hypertension—factors that can be controlled with moderate weight loss and increased physical activity.

Keeping your fasting blood glucose levels below 100 with diet, exercise, and regular monitoring is a good target. Visit the ADA's web site at *www. diabetes.org* for more information.

Types of Diabetes

Below are descriptions of the four general categories of diabetic classification, as outlined by The American Diabetes Association.

Type 1 diabetes: Results from the body's failure to produce insulin, the hormone that "unlocks" the cells of the body, allowing glucose to enter and fuel them. It is estimated that 5-10% of Americans who are diagnosed with diabetes have Type 1 diabetes.

Type 2 diabetes: Results from insulin resistance (a condition in which the body fails to properly use insulin), combined with relative insulin deficiency. Most Americans who are diagnosed with diabetes have Type 2 diabetes.

Gestational diabetes: Immediately after pregnancy, 5% to 10% of women with gestational diabetes are found to have diabetes, usually, Type 2.

Pre-diabetes: Pre-diabetes is a condition that occurs when a person's blood glucose levels are higher than normal, but not high enough for a diagnosis of Type 2 diabetes. There are 57 million Americans who have pre-diabetes, in addition to the 23.6 million with diabetes.

Good Cholesterol vs. Bad Cholesterol

Below are two general descriptions of LDL cholesterol and HDL cholesterol provided by the American Heart Association.

What is LDL cholesterol?

Low-density lipoprotein is the major cholesterol carrier in the blood. If too much LDL cholesterol circulates in the blood, it can slowly build up in the walls of the arteries feeding the heart and brain. Together with other substances it can form plaque, a thick, hard deposit that can clog those arteries (atherosclerosis). A clot (thrombus) that forms near this plaque can block the blood flow to part of the heart muscle and cause a heart attack. If a clot blocks the blood flow to part of the brain, a stroke results. A high level of LDL cholesterol (160 mg/dL and above) reflects an increased risk of heart disease. If you have heart disease, your LDL cholesterol should be less than 100 mg/dL and your doctor may even set your goal to be less than 70 mg/dL. That's why LDL cholesterol is called "bad" cholesterol. Lower levels of LDL cholesterol reflect a lower risk of heart disease.

There is new evidence that elevated levels of LDLs also inhibit fat breakdown. Dr Johan Björkegren and colleagues at the Karolinska Institute in Sweden have found that, "LDL or 'bad' cholesterol inhibits the breakdown of fat in fat cells, thus suggesting that it is a regulator of fat stores. The finding also suggests that drugs, such as statins, which lower LDL cholesterol, may also promote the breakdown of fat stores."

What is HDL cholesterol?

About one-third to one-fourth of blood cholesterol is carried by HDL. Medical experts think HDL tends to carry cholesterol away from the arteries and back to the liver, where it's passed from the body. Some experts believe HDL removes excess cholesterol from plaques and thus slows their growth. HDL cholesterol is known as "good" cholesterol because a high HDL level seems to protect against heart attack. The opposite is also true: a low HDL level (less than 40 mg/dL in men; less than 50 mg/dL in women) indicates a greater risk.

Cholesterol

Cholesterol is a naturally occurring waxy, fatty-substance that circulates throughout all parts of the body. Among other functions, cholesterol assists in the production of cell membranes, hormonal regulation, and in the normal functioning of the nervous system. Its presence is necessary for the body to perform daily activities. Many people make the mistake of eating foods that can cause excessive cholesterol buildup in the arterial walls (known as atherosclerosis), which was discussed in Chapter 1. As fatty plaque builds up, hypertension, coronary artery disease and, ultimately, acute events including heart failure can occur.

Because cholesterol and other fatty substances cannot be dissolved in the blood stream, they are transported to cells by lipoproteins. The American Heart Association focuses on two types of cholesterol (see page 17), both of which are based on the amount of lipoproteins an individual has. Low Density Lipoproteins (LDLs) are generally referred to as the "bad" cholesterol and High Density Lipoproteins (HDLs) are known as the "good" cholesterol.

Total cholesterol/HDL number provides a proven ratio for determining your risk in developing Coronary Heart Disease. Below are normal ranges for cholesterol:

> Total: <200 mg/dL
> LDL: <100 mg/dL
> HDL: >50 mg/dL

Lifestyle Factors

Obesity, BMI, and Waist Circumference

Understanding your body's weight classification is extremely important in developing a healthy lifestyle and can help you to determine whether you are at risk of developing conditions such as metabolic syndrome or cardiovascular disease, which have been linked to excessive body fat.

A study published in the *New England Journal of Medicine* found that, "Having a large waistline can almost double your risk of dying prematurely even if your body mass index is within the 'normal' range." Increases in waist circumference can indicate a greater amount of belly fat, which has been linked to the development of metabolic syndrome and cardiovascular disease.

A quick reference for determining your body weight classification is a measurement known as Body Mass Index (BMI).

How to Find Your BMI and What it Means for Your Health

To determine your BMI (Body Mass Index), use the formula below:

$$BMI = \frac{weight\ (lb) \times 702}{height\ (inches)^2}$$

After you have found your BMI, use that measurement to find where your BMI lies within the guidelines below.

The Center for Disease Control (CDC) provides the following overview of BMI:

An adult who has a BMI of 18.5 or lower is considered underweight.

An adult who has a BMI between 18.5 and 24.9 is considered healthy.

An adult who has a BMI between 25 and 29.9 is considered overweight.

An adult who has a BMI of 30 or higher is considered obese.

While BMI is a useful measurement for determining your body weight classification, it is important to note that, because it does not take into account the fact that muscle weighs more than fat, you should also be sure to utilize additional measurement tools such as waist circumference and body fat skin-fold measurements. Contact your local fitness or medical center to find out how to have these measurements taken.

Stress Response

Dr. Herbert Benson popularized the mind-body approach to medicine and has since pioneered research on the positive effects of relaxation therapy and self-care when dealing with chronic diseases, including heart disease, hypertension, and intestinal discomfort.

The American Medical Student Association defines the mind-body approach as demonstrating "physical, chemical, mental and spiritual interconnectedness, and currently encompasses a wide variety of techniques. These include biofeedback, relaxation training, autogenic training, psycho synthesis, meditation, guided imagery, spiritual healing, prayer, and many other short-term psychotherapeutic interventions."

"To the extent that one's medical condition and/or symptoms are caused or made worse by stress, we can help"
—Herbert Benson, Director Emeritus, Benson-Henry Institute for Mind Body Medicine

So, can our bodies really be affected by our thoughts and stresses? Yes. Stress is a primary risk factor that can lead to hypertension, and ultimately a pro-inflammatory state where your body becomes increasingly susceptible to inflammation. Long-term inflammation can eventually weaken your circulatory system and decrease your body's immune system. Heart disease is not the only chronic disease that can result from an extended pro-inflammatory period—cancer, arthritis, gastrointestinal disease or irritable bowel syndrome, asthma, and Alzheimer's have also been linked to heighted states of inflammation. Stress has also been shown to have a negative impact on cholesterol levels.

Stress, whether good (eustress) or bad (distress), generally can be classified as either short-term or long-term. The Mayo Clinic in Minnesota categorizes stress into acute (short, abrupt response) and chronic (longer, lasting months or years).

Acute Stress: "Acute stress, also known as the fight-or-flight response, is your body's immediate reaction to a threat, challenge or scare. The acute stress response is immediate, it's intense, and in certain circumstances, it can be thrilling. Examples of stressors that may cause an acute stress response are a job interview, a fender bender or an exhilarating ski run."

Chronic Stress: "Chronic stress results from long-term exposure to acute stress. The chronic stress response is much more subtle than is the acute stress response, but the effects may be longer lasting and more problematic. The stressors which may lead to chronic stress are the nagging, day-to-day life situations that often seem unrelenting. Think relationship problems, work difficulties and financial woes."

How Do You Know if You're Stressed Out?

Everyone experiences stress and responds to stress differently. How you handle it depends on your physical and mental health at the time. A situation that places severe stress on you might not have much of an impact on someone else, and vice versa.

We all experience short-term stress once in a while, such as taking a test, giving a speech, or trying something new that make your heart pound or your palms sweat. While you may notice these physical signs during the event, they typically disappear quickly afterwards, usually before resulting in serious health consequences.

There are also those guaranteed stressors like losing a job, getting married, having a baby, getting divorced, changing jobs, buying a house. These types of stressors are usually manageable in the short-term. But you should definitely utilize some stress relieving activities to get you through the rough spots.

One technique for identifying and dealing with your stress is the 3-Step System on page 22. You can also take the Miller & Smith Stress Test (see Appendix A, page 139) to help determine your stress level.

The 3-Step System is particularly useful for acute stress. For long-term or chronic stress, I find journaling works extremely well. Journaling can help you to organize your thoughts, become focused on your long-term goals, and develop strategies to address your stress. Think it and ink it! Once you have a great idea or an important thought, write it out on a piece of paper. Holding thoughts in will cause information overload, leading to a confusion of thought and clarity.

Creating a mind map can be an excellent tool for identifying the various factors contributing to your heart health, which can ultimately help you control these factors and lead a healthier life.

HEALTHY HEART MIND MAP

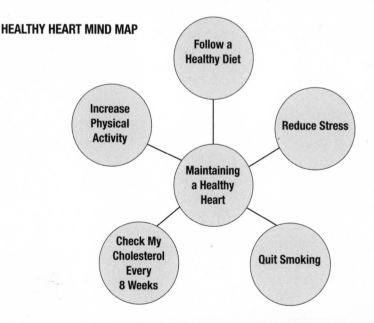

Start out by developing a goal for your heart health. Next, write down any factors you can think of that will help you achieve this goal. Use the sample chart on page 21 to help you develop your own Healthy Heart Mind Map.

3-Step System

We have learned that stress presents itself in multiple forms. In order to control stress, I have developed the *Exercises for Heart Health* 3-Step System that addresses the physiological responses of stress...good or bad.

Step 1: Identify the activity as a stressor and connect with the response.

When your heart rate rises, blood pressure goes up (sense of unsteadiness), and you become hyper alert, chances are you are under a short-term stressor (for example, running across the street)

Step 2: Sit down somewhere quiet.

Find a place that is completely out of the stressor context. For example, a quiet car with the windows up, a park bench, or your living room. Close the blinds if possible, turn the background noise off, and stick your phone in drawer! Basically, find somewhere quiet where you can remove yourself from the stressful situation you are experiencing.

Step 3: Deep breathing and full body contraction.

Sit down, tighten your toes and hands as much as possible, and hold this position for 5 seconds. You will begin to feel your entire body contract. Release your contraction and imagine your body melting into the chair with your jaw dropping and your mouth opening wide. Hold this position for another 5 Seconds and then take 5 deep breaths into your middle back and lower ribs. Complete this series three times. It should take you about 1 minute.

Sleep

Many of us do not give much thought to how much sleep we're getting and how our sleeping patterns can affect our bodies. However, it is important for you to discuss with your physician any sleep disorders you may have. Lack of sleep has been shown to contribute to weight gain, lower immune system function, slower recovery from exercise sessions, and decreased neuro-cognitive function (specifically short and long term memory).

Individuals who consistently fail to get enough sleep have also been shown to exhibit increased stress levels, compromised metabolism and insulin resistance, which is needed to regulate blood sugar levels in the blood (*Experience Magazine,* November 2008). Consistent lack of sleep gradually accumulates a chronic deficit within the body. Dr. Alexandros N. Vgontzas, M.D., director of the Sleep Research and Treatment Center at Penn State University states, "If you lose one night of sleep, your mental performance is like you're legally drunk. We've seen this effect in people who reduce their sleep from eight hours to six."

"Depression and heart disease seem to be intertwined...You can't treat the heart in isolation from the patient's mental health."
— Judith H. Lichtman of Yale University of School of Public Health

As shown in a study done by Dr. Stuart F. Quan, M.D. of Harvard Medical School, severe sleep disorders such as sleep apnea have also been linked to weight gain and changes in blood chemistries. Dr. Quan's team noted the "Patients with severe sleep disordered breathing consumed significantly more fat, cholesterol, saturated fat, and protein compared with individuals who had less disturbed sleep." In turn, individuals with such severe sleep disorders are also at higher risk of developing cardiovascular disease, hypertension, and stroke.

Mental Health and Heart Disease
Many years of research has proven that increasing one's physical activity can help to improve a variety of diseases, most notably improvements in cardiovascular function. A well-balanced exercise program, such as the one in this book, can also greatly improve your psychological health, specifically in the case of various depressive states.

Because cardiac procedures can bring about significant changes in a patient's outlook on life, many cardiac rehabilitation programs screen for signs of depression following heart surgery. Signs of post-traumatic stress and depressive-like symptoms are commonly reported after such invasive procedures, so pre- and post-operative counseling should always accompany cardiac procedures.

In 2008, Dr. Mary Whooley, M.D. published a study which investigated the connection between physical activity and depression. She found that "cardiac patients who had symptoms of depression had a 31% higher rate of cardiovascular events. Moreover, with coronary heart disease patients, depression may be associated with worse outcomes, primarily because it tends to curtail physical activity." While it may not seem very encouraging to know that depression can increase one's risk of cardiovascular problems, Dr. Whooley's study also found that exercise training can improve both depressive symptoms and markers of cardiovascular risk (*Journal of the American Medical Association*, 2008).

CHAPTER FOUR

The Path to Better Health

The Benefits of Exercise

The rewards of exercise—from preventing chronic health conditions to boosting confidence and self esteem—are hard to ignore. And these benefits are yours for the taking, regardless of age, sex or physical ability. If you still need more convincing, consider that exercise has proven time and time again that if there is indeed an "anti-aging pill," physical activity is the answer. *Exercises for Heart Health* uses a safe and effective circuit-based approach that develops overall work capacity, stamina, and movement.

Benefits of Exercise

Before getting into the specifics of the *Exercises for Heart Health* program I find it vitally important to explain the general health benefits of a structured strength training program.

Harvard Medical School has developed a very helpful and informative guide on the benefits of exercise, specifically related to strength training. Their original guide was later reprinted in the larger special report "Strength and Power Training: A Special Health Report from Harvard Medical School".

This report notes the following benefits of a fitness program that utilizes strength training, and its benefits for improving cardiovascular function:

1. . Strong muscles pluck oxygen and nutrients from the blood much more efficiently than weak ones. That means any activity requires less cardiac effort and puts less strain on your heart.
2. Strong muscles are better at sopping up sugar in the blood and helping the body stay sensitive to insulin (which helps cells remove sugar from the blood).
3. Strong muscles enhance weight control and decrease stress on joints.
4. Weak muscles accelerate the loss of independence and mobility, both of which are extremely important in daily tasks such as grocery shopping, getting out of bed, walking up your steps, or helping your neighbor cut that pesky tree branch.

So now that Harvard has assisted in defining several proven benefits related to heart and total body health, let's speak to the specific guidelines you should follow in your daily *Exercises for Heart Health* program.

Exercise Categories

This book's exercise program is broken down into three primary categories:
1. **Stability**
2. **Stamina**
3. **Movement**

Stability
Stability training teaches the body to stabilize your hips, back, and shoulders. We then apply strength exercises like squats or lunges, called resistance training.

Core Stability
Core training has gotten a lot of press since the mid-nineties, when greater awareness of the importance of such training began to take hold. Core strength, the result of core training, should more appropriately be named core stability.

Forward bending and backward extensions occur in what is called a sagittal plane of motion. Examples of common exercises that occur in this plane are toe touches and back extensions, both of which are dynamic movements.

26

Planes of the Body

Sagittal Plane (Lateral Plane)
A vertical plane running from front to back; divides the body or any of its parts into right and left sides.

Coronal Plane (Frontal Plane)
A vertical plane running from side to side; divides the body or any of its parts into anterior and posterior portions.

Transverse Plane (Axial Plane)
A horizontal plane; divides the body or any of its parts into upper and lower parts.

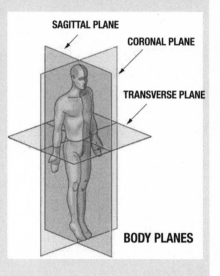

SAGITTAL PLANE
CORONAL PLANE
TRANSVERSE PLANE
BODY PLANES

Stamina
Stamina focuses on building the energy systems of the body, and involves maintaining energy and strength for a long period of time while performing a particular activity. *Exercises for Heart Health* works on building your total work capacity (functional capacity) by changing rest intervals, and incorporating circuits and functional exercises such as walking up and down stairs or picking up objects.

Developing endurance or stamina and work capacity are two primary goals of *Exercises for Heart Health*. Endurance is broken down into two types, cardio respiratory and muscular. These are defined by the Centers for Disease Control as follows:

Cardio Respiratory Endurance
Cardio respiratory endurance is the ability of the body's circulatory and respiratory systems to supply fuel during sustained physical activity (US-DHHS, 1996 as adapted from Corbin & Lindsey, 1994). To improve your cardio respiratory endurance, try activities that keep your heart rate elevated at a safe level for a sustained length of time such as walking, swimming, or bicycling. The activity you choose does not have to be strenuous to improve

your cardio respiratory endurance. Start slowly with an activity you enjoy, and gradually work up to a more intense pace.

Muscular Endurance

Muscular endurance is the ability of the muscle to continue to perform without fatigue (USDHHS, 1996 as adapted from Wilmore & Costill, 1994). To improve your muscular endurance, try cardio respiratory activities such as walking, jogging, bicycling, or dancing.

Walking

The old adage, 'an apple a day keeps the doctor away' might still be the case, but recent studies have indicated that 'a walk a day keeps the doctor away!'

Starting an outdoor walking program is the most cost effective way to access regular exercise, whether you go for a power walk or take a leisurely stroll. Walking is one of the best exercises and can reduce the risk of many diseases as well as clear your mind of the stressors of the day.

The purpose of any good fitness program is to allow you to perform activities of daily life with ease and enjoyment. Walking can be safely integrated using soft walking trails, grassy fields, or well-kept tracks. I believe walking to be an extremely safe and effective method of using your entire body as it is a practical way to apply the core and strength exercises I teach in this book.

Movement

Movement consists of flexibility training, soft tissue rolling, and balance training.

The movement section of exercises focuses on increasing body temperature, improving body awareness, enhancing coordination, and self-applied soft tissue therapy. A recent *New York Times* article entitled "Stretching: The Truth" discusses the benefits of movement-based exercises for increasing overall functional capabilities.

The article notes, "A well-designed warm-up starts by increasing body heat and blood flow. Warm muscles and dilated blood vessels pull oxygen from the bloodstream more efficiently and use stored muscle fuel more effectively. They also withstand loads better. One significant if gruesome study found that the leg-muscle tissue of laboratory rabbits could be stretched farther before ripping if it had been electronically stimulated—that is, warmed up."

Benefits of Walking

- **Manages your weight.** Combined with healthy eating, physical activity is key to long-lasting weight control. Keeping your weight within healthy limits can lower your risks of Type 2 diabetes, heart disease, stroke, cancer, sleep apnea, and osteoarthritis.

- **Controls your blood pressure.** Physical activity strengthens the heart, so it can pump more blood with less effort and with less pressure on the arteries. Staying fit is just as effective as some medications in keeping blood pressure levels low.

- **Decreases your risk of heart attack.** Exercise, such as brisk walking for three hours a week, or just half an hour a day, is associated with a 30% to 40% lower risk of heart disease in women. (Based on the NIH's 20-year Nurses' Health Study of 72,000 female nurses.)

- **Boosts "good" cholesterol (high-density lipoproteins or HDL).** Physical activity helps reduce low-density lipoproteins (LDL or "bad" cholesterol) in the blood, which can cause plaque buildup along the artery walls, a major cause of heart attacks.

- **Lowers your risk of stroke.** Regular, moderate exercise equivalent to brisk walking for an hour a day, five days a week, can cut the risk of stroke in half, according to a Harvard study of more than 11,000 men.

- **Reduces your risk of breast cancer and Type 2 diabetes.** The Nurses' Health Study also links regular activity to risk reductions for both of these diseases. In another study, people at high risk of diabetes cut their risk in half by combining consistent exercise, like walking, with lower fat intake and a 5% to 7% weight loss.

- **Reduces need for gallstone surgery.** Regular walking or other physical activity lowers the risk of needing gallstone surgery by 20% to 31%, found a Harvard study of more than 60,000 women ages 40 to 65.

- **Protects against hip fracture.** Consistent activity diminishes the risk of hip fracture, concludes a study of more than 30,000 men and women ages 20 to 93.

- **Other studies have suggested a daily brisk walk can also help prevent depression, colon cancer, osteoporosis, and impotence.**

In addition, walks may lengthen lifespan, lower stress levels, relieve arthritis and back pain, strengthen muscles, bones and joint, improve sleep, and elevate mood and sense of well-being.

How could you go wrong with walking once a day? Try it for two weeks and keep a journal about where you walk and how you feel before/after the walk. Make note of your fitness level before the two weeks, and afterwards.

Remember to keep a steady routine by walking for at least 30 minutes a day, five or more days a week to get the most out of your program. Consult your doctor first before starting any exercise program!

Make the walks fun too—bring a friend, walk your dog, or listen to music.

(Contributed by Angela Pappano, MS, NCC and UC Berkeley Women's Health letter)

How the Exercises Were Chosen

Exercises for Heart Health is a simple system that I have developed for you to use in your day-to-day life. This system has been applied through years of patients, clients, and training sessions and has been shown to be highly effective at improving functional activities.

Guidelines are as follows:

1. **Quality not quantity:** You will be given a beginner, intermediate, advanced, and maintenance program. There is an optional preparatory program to build your stamina and function if this is your first dedicated effort to exercising regularly. Developing correct technique through properly executed exercises is the most important aspect of any exercise program.
2. **Less is better than more:** When in doubt do less! You can always add additional sets, reps, and exercises later in your program design.
3. **Consistency is a habit:** A habit is something you do without thinking twice. It is said that a habit can take 21-25 days to form. Challenge yourself to engage in daily approaches to heart health that you feel confident in. Following the exercise program is great, but adding leisure activities like gardening, stretching for 15 minutes, meditating, or taking a qigong class

at the community center are all examples of engaging your health on a daily basis. Health will be a habit and thus a lifestyle, not an effort. Enjoy what you do.

By following the above elements, the exercises in this book provide a convenient, cost-effective opportunity to alleviating the side effects of poor heart health. **Remember—in maintaining a healthy heart, consistency is key to overall success.**

CHAPTER FIVE

Rules of the Road

Exercise Precautions

Basic Exercise Guidelines

In August 2007, the American College of Sports Medicine and the American Heart Association released a new series of recommendations for physical activity guidelines geared towards healthy populations. Below are highlights:

- **Build your activity levels slowly and progressively over time.** Utilizing the guidance of a fitness professional should be considered.
- **Strengthening and stretching muscles can take stress off of joints with arthritis pain**.
- **Break up the amount of time you work out.** Instead of performing 30 minutes of continuous exercise, utilize shorter 10-15 minute segments of swimming, biking, and strength development. Consistency and quality of technique in movements are paramount, quantity can be increased. Work up to 4-6 days per week of moving your body with 45 minutes to1 hour of continuous activity as your goal.

- **Fall prevention has become a very important aspect of fitness programming.** Exercises that utilize balance, coordination, and multitasking (e.g. catching a ball while standing on one leg) are becoming more common. Creating confidence in one's movement capabilities leads to greater independence and improved quality of life on a daily basis.
- **The body learns through movement, not isolation.** Multi-joint exercises such as squatting, dead lifts, pulling, rotational patterns, and extension (spidermans, on page 100, for example) teaches muscles to work together, ultimately increasing stability of the joints in a more effective way. For example, the muscles in the front and back of the leg (quad/hamstring, respectively) are both working when standing on one leg, hence creating greater coordination between the lower body muscles.

Cardiovascular Health Physical Activity Guidelines

I am regularly asked the question: If I have risk factors that could potentially be detrimental to the health of my heart, yet want to exercise, what guidelines should I follow?

The American College of Sports Medicine (ACSM) and American Heart Association recently updated joint exercise guideline recommendations for physical activity. Now included in those are balance and flexibility training along with the traditional aerobic activity and balanced nutrition recommendations (Visit *www.americanheart.org* or *www.acsm.org* for more information).

Tips for Leading a More Active Lifestyle with CVD

Below you will find a quick list of highlights from the American College of Sports Medicine for people with cardiovascular disease and how they can increase their overall activity levels.

1. Consistent, regular aerobic exercise lowers heart rate and blood pressure at rest and at any given level of exercise. This decreases the workload on the heart.

   Comment: Progressively building up your body's ability to adapt to the physical demands of exercise allows for long-term positive outcomes. This is the called the progressive overload theory.

2. Exercise increases the ability to take in and utilize oxygen, making the body more efficient during activities of daily living. This decreases

the overall stress upon the cardiovascular system, enabling prolonged activities with greater ease.

Comment: Activities of daily living, including shopping, gardening, mowing the lawn, or walking up and down steps all have caloric and oxygen demands based upon their energy requirements. Larger muscles combined with lengthier efforts require larger amounts of work from the body. Couple these two elements with increased intensity (i.e. walking intensely for an hour versus at a leisurely pace), naturally requires more work from the body.

3. How often should I exercise? Three to four times a week for 12 weeks or more is a good initial goal. Re-assessment should follow to reinforce technique, gains, and program design.

Comment: Periodically re-assessing your progress helps to determine if you are making progress, so you can adjust your program.

4. How much should I exercise per session? 30-60 minutes is optimum.

Comment: Throughout Exercises for Heart Health, *we want you to be active consistently yet also balance structured exercise with leisure activities. Shoot for three times a week of structured moderate-higher level activity, and two to three times a week of leisurely low-moderate activity.*

5. Single-set circuits provide an effective stimulus for the heart. Large muscle movements involving exercises such as squatting, lifting, pulling, pushing, and pressing are ideal.

Comment: Quality vs. Quantity. Doing more in the initial stages of the exercise program (i.e. multiple sets) does not equal quality. Single set circuits done with less rest between sets is preferable in the beginner stage, an extra set can be added later on.

6. 10-15 repetition range is optimum.

Comment: This repetition range will stimulate physiological and anatomical changes necessary for the proper cardiac program foundation.

7. 5-6 hours/week provides an adequate stimulus to achieve introductory to intermediate levels of fitness and overall sense of well-being.

Comment: Enjoying activities as a part of life will create greater compliance and adherence to healthier living. Both are concerns in people with high risk profiles.

8. Balance, flexibility, soft tissue (foam rolling) body work should also be considered.

Comment: Comprehensive fitness program should be just that, comprehensive and fun. Adding new fitness elements to your program will keep you engaged.

9. Increase your overall movement time through exercise and leisure activities. Leisure activities include golfing, gardening, and moderate-paced walking.

Comment: Leisure activities are the easiest and least intrusive lifestyle modification that can be made. Find an activity you enjoy and try it at least once a week. Find activities that use multi-joints and large muscle groups.

Exercise Essentials Checklist

Exercise Preparation

✓ **Exercise Location:** Is your environment safe, clean, and free of debris?

✓ **Proper Footwear:** Are you wearing proper athletic footwear?

✓ **Comfortable Athletic Wear:** Do you have clothes that allow freedom of movement?

✓ **Hydration:** Be sure to drink 6 glasses of fluid over the course of your day.

Exercise Equipment

- Broomstick
- Rolled up towel
- Mirror
- Dumbbells
- Therabands (you can also work with a partner if you don't have a Theraband)
- Physio-ball: Inflate the ball to the point where you can press your thumb on the surface without it sinking in.
- Tennis ball or racquet ball

Playing it Safe: Important Safety Precautions

- **Body Positioning:** Brace your core, achieve proper alignment, feel the placement of your feet, and always move first from your core before moving your limbs
- **Keep a Heart Health Journal:** In this journal, you can record how you're feeling on any given day and what activities you did during that time. You should also record what kinds of exercises you did on each

day and how you felt during and after your exercise session. Keeping track of this information will help you better understand your own health, which is a crucial step on the road to recovery.

- **Rate of Perceived Exertion (RPE):** You can use the chart below to gauge how hard you are working during your session. The corresponding numerical values may also be helpful for you to record in your Heart Health Journal, if you choose to keep one.

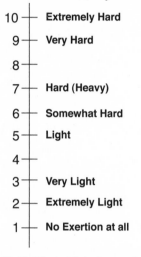

10 — Extremely Hard

9 — Very Hard

8 —

7 — Hard (Heavy)

6 — Somewhat Hard

5 — Light

4 —

3 — Very Light

2 — Extremely Light

1 — No Exertion at all

- **Talk Test:** This is another useful way of determining how hard you are working. As you are exercising, gauge how easily you are able to converse and use the guidelines below to figure out the intensity of your exertion.

    If you can carry on a normal conversation while exercising, you are likely working **aerobically**, which means your body is using oxygen as it's primary energy source. If you can work aerobically for up to 30-45 minutes, your body will also be using fat as an energy source, which is an excellent foundation for building your exercise program.

    Anaerobic work, characterized below as medium intensity, should be introduced 8 weeks into your exercise program. Examples include hill walking, bike sprints, etc. When performing anaerobic exercise, you may notice your leg muscles starting to feel a bit tight, your chest will expand, you will begin to sweat, and your heart rate will reach about 40-50 beats above your resting heart rate (see page 39 for more details on determining your heart rate).

    – *Low Intensity:* Complete sentences, breathing rate normal

    – *Medium Intensity:* Broken sentences, breathing rate slightly labored

    – *High Intensity:* Cannot converse, breathing rate labored

- **Be sure to see your healthcare provider regularly for check-ups**
- **Determining your heart rate:** To determine your heart rate, place the tips of your index, second and third fingers on your wrist, below the base of your thumb. You can also place the tips of your index and second fingers on your neck, along either side of your windpipe. During exercise, it is recommended that you find your pulse on your wrist, rather than on your neck.

  While pressing lightly with your fingers, you should be able to feel your pulse. If you don't feel your pulse, move your fingers around slightly until you find your pulse.

  Watch the second hand of a clock or watch and count the number of beats you feel in 10 seconds. Using that number, you can calculate your heart rate with the formula below:

  (Beats in ten seconds) x 6 = (Heart Rate)

Adults over 18 years of age typically have a resting heart rate of 60-100 beats per minute. To better understand your own heart rate, you should check your pulse before, and immediately after, you exercise. This will give you a better idea of what your body normally does at rest, and to what level your heart should be working during an exercise session.

Important Assessments

Fitness programs designed for persons with a history of heart problems can provide an important service that improves quality of life and function for a wide group of people. For those beginning exercise for the first time, or that haven't exercised in quite some time, it's recommended they be assessed by their medical practitioner.

Below are basic assessments that should be considered:

- **Medical Tests**

  Medical tests include blood panels, neurological/reflexive tests, updated family history, stress test, etc. These are tests that your medical provider can provide based upon his/her clinical assessment of health and risk profile. Open dialogue with your medical practitioner, particularly if you have a history of heart problems, is paramount.

- **Fitness Tests (Functional and Physical Assessments)**
  - *Functional Assessment:* The Functional Assessment will provide you with a direct measurement of how you can improve in your activities of daily living. This includes walking stairs, getting in and out of chairs, etc. Refer to Chapter 7, page 136 for the Functional Assessment.

Calculating Target Heart Rate

Your target heart rate is the level of exertion you should aim for when exercising in order to gain the most benefits from your workout. Your target heart rate is also a useful range for how your body is responding to your workout.

Target heart rate is 60-80% of your maximum heart rate, depending on what level of exertion you wish to work at.

Different Training Zones

Below is a list of the different levels of exertion and the corresponding percentage you would use to target heart rate:

Recovery Zone - 60% to 70%

Active recovery training should fall into this zone (ideally at the lower end). It's also useful for very early pre-season and closed season cross training when the body needs to recover and replenish.

Aerobic Zone - 70% to 80%

Exercising in this zone will help to develop your aerobic system and, in particular, your ability to transport and utilize oxygen. Continuous or rhythmic endurance training, like running and hiking, should fall under this heart rate zone.

Anaerobic Zone – 80% to 90%

Training in this zone will help to improve your body's ability to deal with lactic acid. It may also help to increase your lactate threshold.

To determine your target heart rate, you can use the formulas below to calculate your maximum heart rate, and to then find your target heart rate.

220 – age = maximum heart rate
Maximum heart rate x training % = target heart rate

For example, if a 50 year old woman wishes to train at 70% of her maximum heart rate, she would use the below calculations:

220 – 50 = 170
170 x 70% = 119

She would thus aim to reach a heart rate of 117 during her exercise in order to work at her target heart rate.

You can also use the Karvonen Formula, which is based on both maximum heart rate and resting heart. Visit *www.sport-fitness-advisor.com/heart-rate-reserve.html* for more information.

- *Physical Assessment:* The Physical Assessment will provide you with a direct measurement of the improvements you can make in gaining strength as a result of following the exercises in this book. Refer to Chapter 7, page 136 for the Physical Assessment.
- *Waist Size:* To determine your waist-to-height ratio, simply divide your waist size by your height (in inches). A waist-to-height ratio under 50% is generally considered healthy.
- *Stamina:* The average person should be able to walk up a flight of stairs or walk once around an outdoor track without becoming out of breath.
  - **12-Minute Walking Test**
    Find a measured distance, such as a track, and see how much distance you can cover in 12 minutes. Make sure you challenge yourself, while still being able to carry on intermittent conversation with a partner (see the Talk Test on page 37).
    Referring to the Rating of Perceived Exertion (RPE) scale on page 37, you should aim to work at around 5-6 during the first two or three times of repeating this test. Thereafter, challenge yourself to reach a 7-8 on the RPE scale.
  - **Quarter Mile Timed Test**
    Find a measured 400-meter or quarter-mile track. See how long it takes you to cover the specified distance. Aim to work at a 6-7 on the Rate of Perceived Exertion (RPE) scale.
- *Strength:* As you perform the Strength Circuits (see page 129-130), make note of any improvements you have made. For instance, are you able to perform more reps, or have you continued from beginner to intermediate exercises?
- *Flexibility:* Because levels of flexibility can differ greatly from one individual to the next, it is impossible to provide an average measurement of flexibility. Instead, you should aim to determine what improvements you are making in your Physical Assessment (see page 136) from week to week. This will help you gauge whether you are improving your flexibility based on your body's abilities.

■ **Re-Assessment**
Perform the Functional and Physical Assessments again and compare your new results with your original results to determine how much you have improved in your overall strength and function.

Overhead Squat

eel it Here Hips, Back, Shoulders

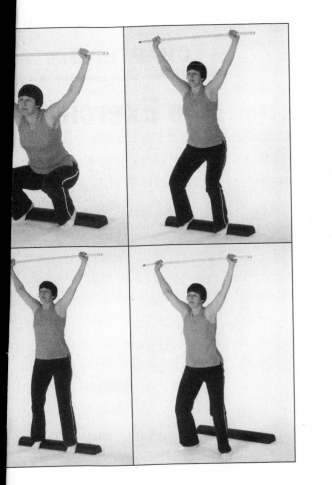

lf with feet hip-width apart. Point your toes to 11 and 1
ns respectively, as this will allow your hips, knees, and
together properly during the squatting movement. Place
mstick) on the crown of you head so your elbows are at a
e, then press the stick above your head. Place a half roller
ls if you feel your body pitching forward. Drop your hips
ble.

Exercise Phases

- **Preparatory Phase:** This phase lasts from two to four weeks depending on your exercise history. The objective of this phase is to build up regular participation and familiarity with the *Exercises for Heart Health* programming.
- **Beginner Phase:** This phase lasts four to six weeks depending on how your body adapts to the program. The objectives are to build stability and movement function.
- **Intermediate Phase:** This phase lasts four weeks. Challenges you with increasing stamina-based circuits to build up your muscular endurance, with increased emphasis on stability.
- **Advanced Phase:** This phase lasts three to four weeks. During it, you are asked to push yourself, pain-free, through challenging strength circuits. Emphasis is on stability and movement through increased practical application.
- **Maintenance:** This phase allows you to have more fun. Play with the different circuits and bonus routines applying the *Exercises for Heart Health* stability, movement, and stamina philosophy.

SET-UP
Position yourse
o'clock positio
ankles to move
the dowel (bro
90-degree angl
under your hee
as low as possi

Stair Walking

Feel it Here Back

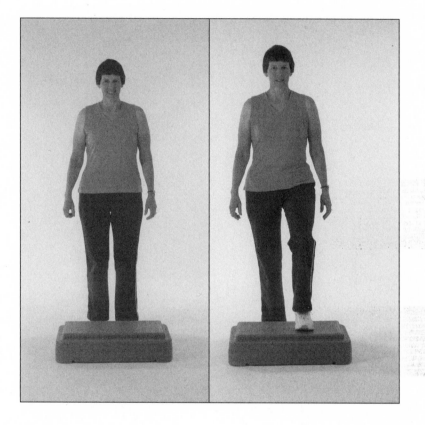

SET-UP

Position yourself in front of a step or set of stairs with feet hip-width apart. Place one foot on the first step. Press the foot into the step to engage your hip and lower back muscles. Use the railing until you get stronger. Feel the full foot pressing into the step without letting the hips slide to the side.

Getting up from a Chair

Feel it Here Core

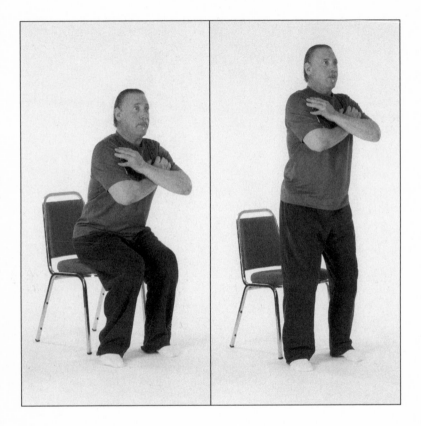

SET-UP

Position yourself on the edge of a chair. Hips should be parallel, or slightly above, knee level. Brace your core and press your feet into the ground.

Standing with Eyes Closed

Feel it Here Fully Body

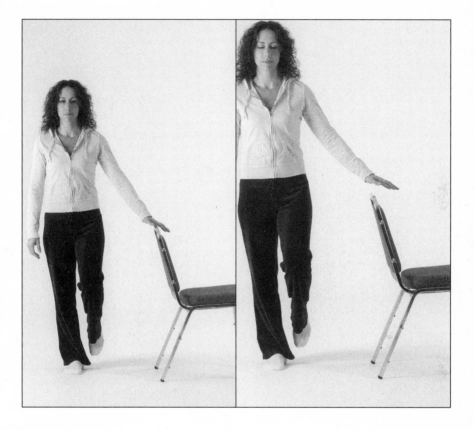

SET-UP

Stand with your feet hip width apart. You should stand near a wall or part-ner for safety. For the two -legged test, rest you hands at your side and close your eyes. With both feet on the ground feel a natural sway similar to a tree in the wind. For the one legged test, close your eyes once your foot is off the ground. With one foot on the ground the sway will increase dramatically with your body wanting to make very quick readjustments to stabilize.

Getting up from the Ground

Feel it Here Core, Shoulders, Legs

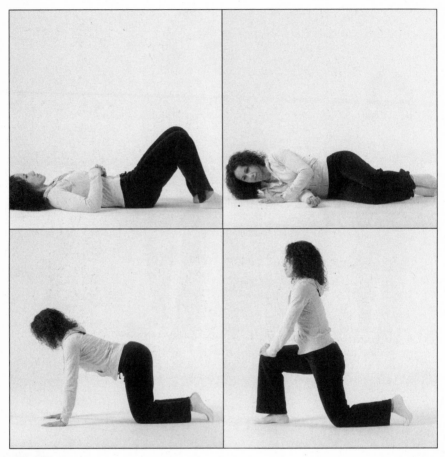

SET-UP

Position yourself on your back or stomach, with your hands above your shoulders. Brace your stomach first, then move your torso and naturally allow your body segments to follow into an all fours position. You should be near a wall or couch if you need assistance getting up.

Heel to Toe Walking

Feel it Here Core, Sides of Legs, Back

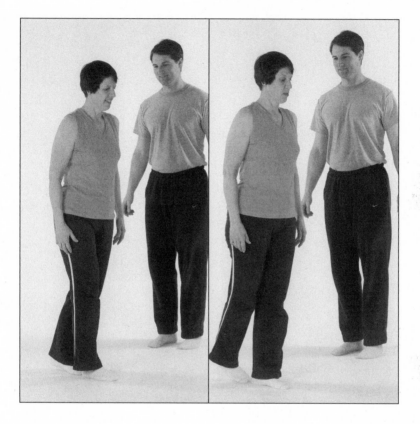

SET-UP
Find a wall or fixed surface prior to beginning this exercise in case you become off balance. Begin with your arms out to the side for added stability. Pick a spot in front of you for focus and begin the movement by placing one foot in front of the other. Experience your upper body attempting to stabilize itself more than when you are in a normal walking position. A dramatic change in stability will occur with one foot in front or behind the other. Take your time and concentrate on the placement of each foot. Repeat backwards toe-to-heel.

Standing Tail Wag

Feel it Here Hips, Lower Spine

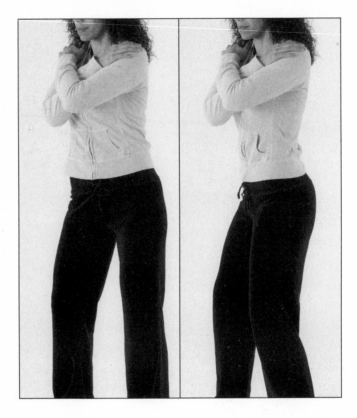

SET-UP

Square your body up facing forward. Cross your hands over your shoulders with your elbows resting on your chest. Keep your head, hips and legs quiet. Keeping your shoulders still, attempt to rotate the hips, without moving any other part of the body. Stay light through your knees.

Chair Sit

Feel it Here Legs

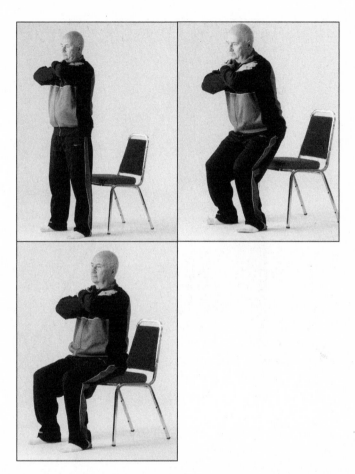

SET-UP

Using the chair as a teaching tool, lower the hips down towards the seat using legs and hips. Hold this position, relax into the chair, repeat. Work on increasing the time held for each rep. A wall can be used if the isometric squat is too much. Position your body against a wall. Walk your hips down the wall by walking your feet out in front of your body. Keep your hips, knees, and toes in line. Maintaining head, shoulder, and tailbone contact with the wall, hold the squatting position as if sitting in a chair. You should not feel pain in your knees. If you do, walk the feet out farther. Breathe into your lower body.

Push-up

Feel it Here Stomach, Chest, Arms, Legs

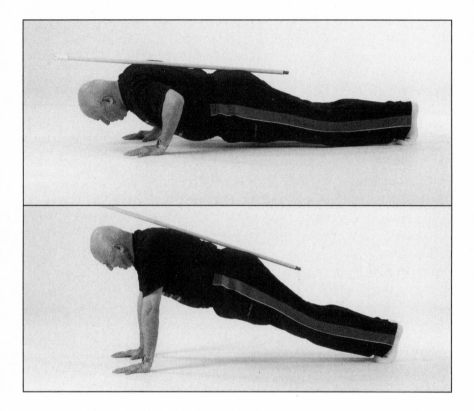

SET-UP

Position yourself on your stomach. Your hands should be parallel to your shoulders. Place a dowel stick along the spine so contact is made with your head and sacrum. Begin the movement by bracing your stomach. Push your toes and hands into the floor, then attempt to press your body away from the floor until your elbows are straight. You should feel your shoulder blades come together as you return to your starting position.

Lateral Plank

Feel it Here Shoulders, Ribs, Obliques, Hip

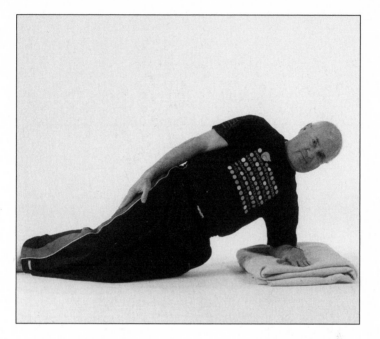

SET-UP

Position you body on one side, on your elbow and hip. Contract the side of your stomach and elevate your hip into alignment with the shoulders and knees.

Lifting Technique

Feel it Here Legs, Stomach, Spine, Shoulders, and Arms.

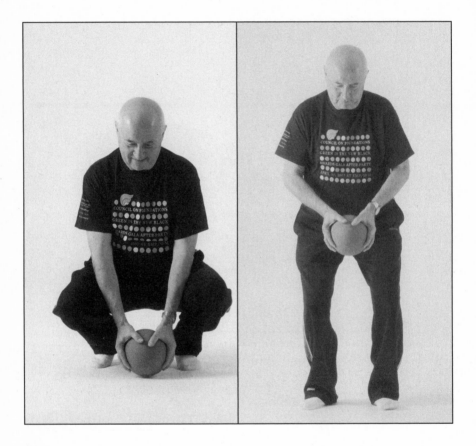

SET-UP

Point your toes to the 11 and 1 o'clock positions. Bend at the hips, knees, and ankles. Keep the object close to your body during the entire motion. Prior to beginning the upward (lifting) movement, brace your stomach and press your feet into the ground, then stand up straight. If you are unable to keep your heels down, it is especially important that you brace your stomach throughout this movement.

Rolling Technique from Floor

Feel it Here Core, Spine, Hips, Back

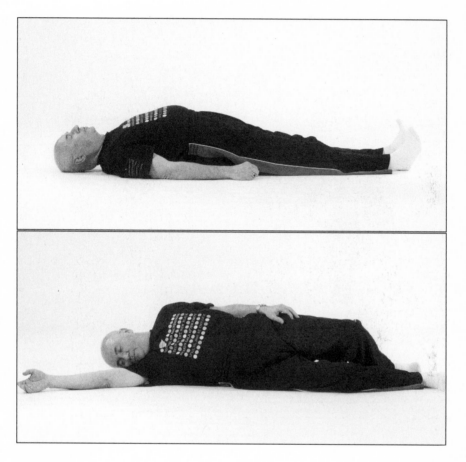

SET-UP

Position yourself on your back. Feel relaxed throughout your body prior to movement. Transition your body into a side-lying position by resting your head on the bottom arm. Rotate your shoulders then the spine, followed by the hips and legs. Rotating first through the spine allows you to maintain better control of your spine.

Ribs Heavy

Feel it Here Lower Ribs, Abs

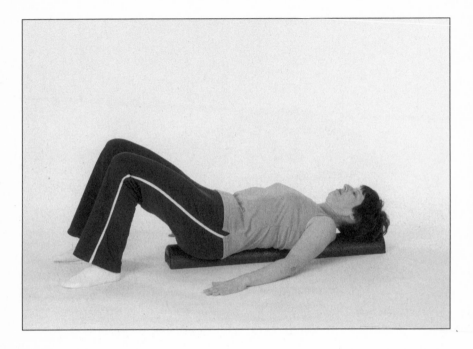

SET-UP

Use a foam roller or towel rolled up lengthwise. Make sure your head, middle back, and hips are in contact with the roller or towel. Feel your lower ribs make contact with the roller, yet make sure you have space in your lower back. This movement replaces pushing your lower back into the ground or flattening out your lower back during core movements, and will be applied to all exercises. When lying on your back, the body should contact the floor at your head, shoulders, hips, upper legs and calves. Your neck, lower back, and space behind your knees should be off the floor.

Hip Hinging

Feel it Here Lower Spine, Hamstrings,

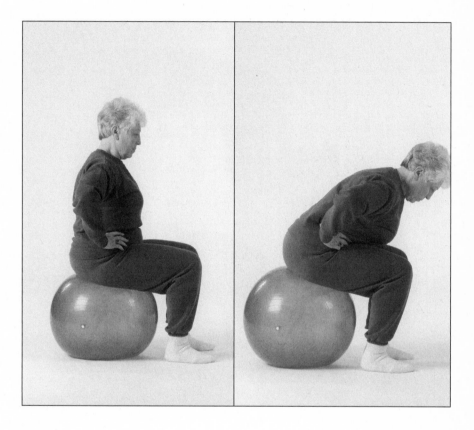

SET-UP

Start the squatting movement from your hips, letting the other parts follow. Feel your upper body positioned over the upper thighs as you bend during the downward motion. Brace your stomach, then begin the upward movement by pressing your feet into the floor, followed by pushing your hips through. For added help with stability, place a broomstick along your spine. Contact should be felt on the back of your head, middle back and tailbone.

Spinal Whip

Feel it Here Middle Back

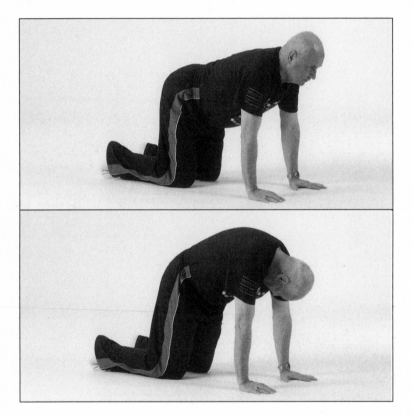

SET-UP

Begin on all fours or standing with your hands on your knees. Rotate from the shoulder blades as they move to the outside of the upper body. Emphasize moving from the middle back through the sternum.

Childs Pose
with Arm Rotation and Lift

Feel it Here Shoulders, Middle Back, Outside Ribs

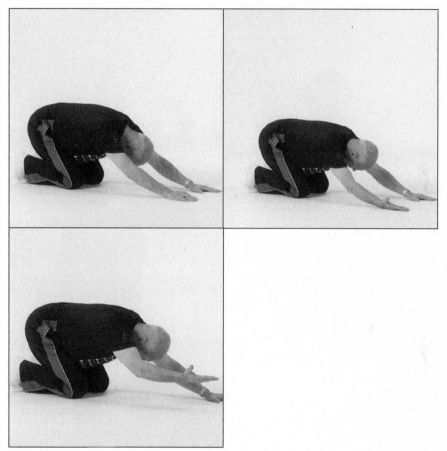

SET-UP

Begin on all fours. Drop your hips back between the legs. Once in a comfortable position, roll your shoulders out and allow the elbows and palms to follow. Attempt the pose with one arm, and then with both arms together.

Standard Lunge

Feel it Here Stomach, Obliques

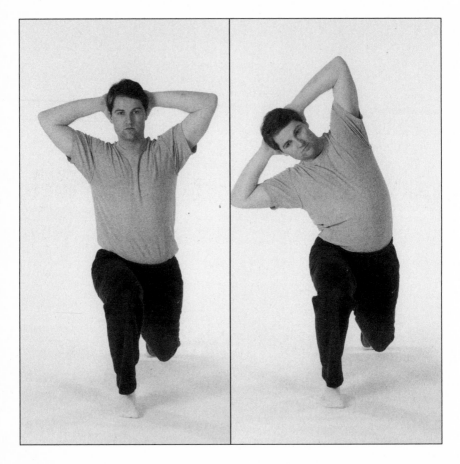

SET-UP

Lunging is nothing more than an exaggerated step. For an advanced lunge (shown, right), make sure your hips are stable and then flex your trunk to the front leg side.

Physio-ball Roll

Feel it Here Stomach, Ribs, Chest, Shoulders

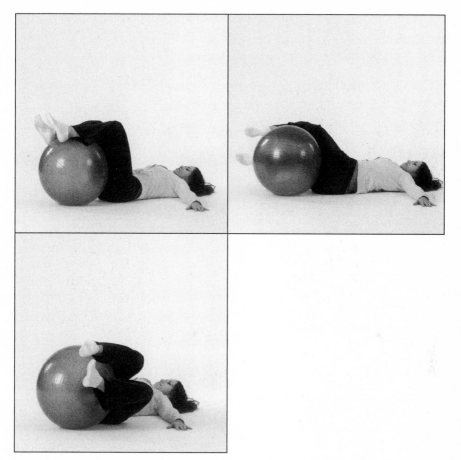

SET-UP

Cup your legs over a Physio-ball at an angle slightly greater than 90 degrees, or a square angle at the knees and hips. Position your arms out to the side with palms down to aid in stability during lower body movement. On the way toward the floor, breathe in and gently press the back of your legs into the ball thereby slowing the legs down. On the way back to your starting position, breathe out and press your hand into the floor to activate the stomach and shoulders. This stabilizes your spine prior to moving the ball.

Thoracic Flex on Roller

Feel it Here Middle Spine, Abdominals

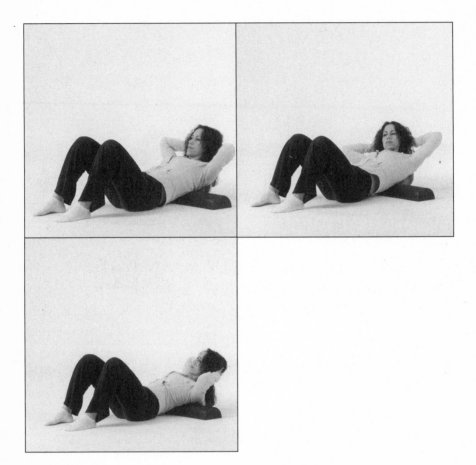

SET-UP

You can use a full roller, half roller, or thick, rolled up towel. Position the roller immediately below your shoulder blades. Your elbows should be pointed to the sides. Feel the foam roller pressing against your middle spine. Keep your ribs heavy (see page 56) into the ground so the core muscles are active and working through the entire motion. Your front abs will be working the entire time but the latter muscles, namely the obliques, are the actual movers.

Bent Knee Hamstring

Feel it Here Back of Upper/Middle Leg

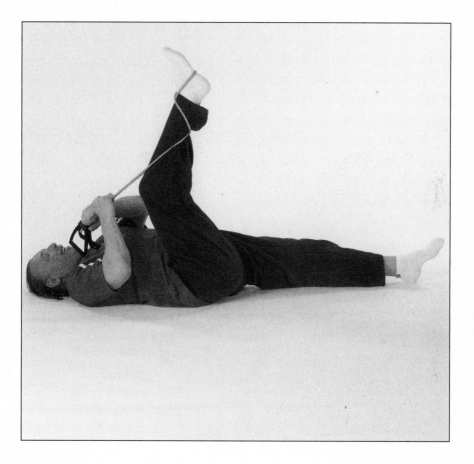

SET-UP

Lay on your back and draw one knee into your chest. Wrap the towel or stretch cord around the arch of your foot. Pull your ankle toward the back of your hip without letting your hip move. Hold the pressure for five seconds. Release and breathe out slowly. Repeat the movement from the newly obtained position.

Adductors with Band

Feel it Here Inner Groin, Hip

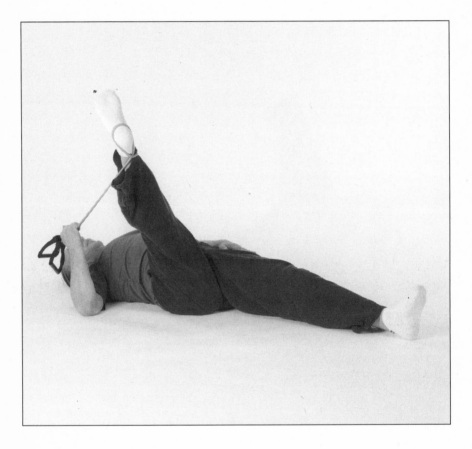

SET-UP

Wrap the towel or stretch cord around the ankle of the leg you want to stretch. Keeping the non-stretching leg down on the floor, press your ankle in toward your body against resistance, and release. Hold the pressure for five seconds. Release and breathe out slowly. Repeat the movement from the newly obtained position.

Abductors

Feel it Here Outer Hip, Obliques, Lower Back

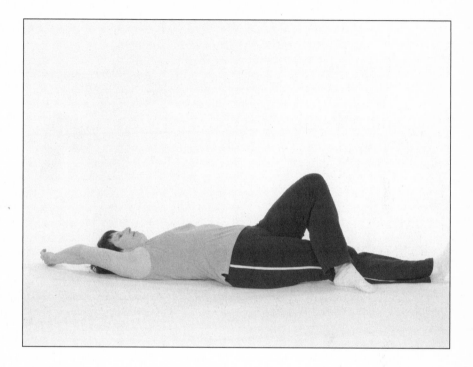

SET-UP

Keeping the non-stretching leg down on the floor, cross the opposite ankle over the leg, pressing against the knee. Hold the pressure for five seconds. Release and breathe out slowly. Repeat the movement from the newly obtained position.

Hip Lifters

Feel it Here Hips, Back

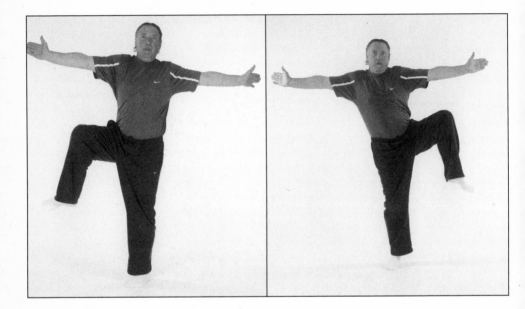

SET-UP

With hands out to the side, draw the hip out and knee up behind the arm.
Feel the hips and back working throughout this exercise.

Windshield Washer

Feel it Here Inner Hip Joints

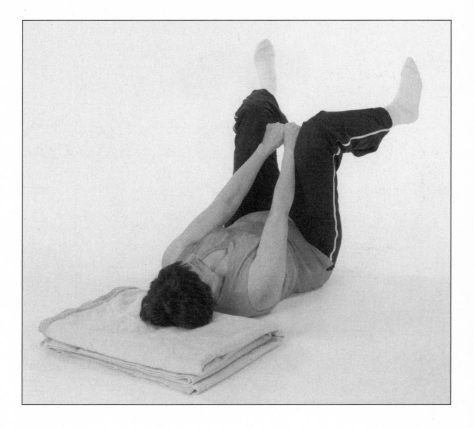

SET-UP

Lay on your back. Squeeze a ball or double fists between your knees. Position your head on a towel to take stress off your neck and arms. Maintain pressure on the object while rotating your hips inward.

Roll and Hold

Feel it Here Upper and Lower Spine

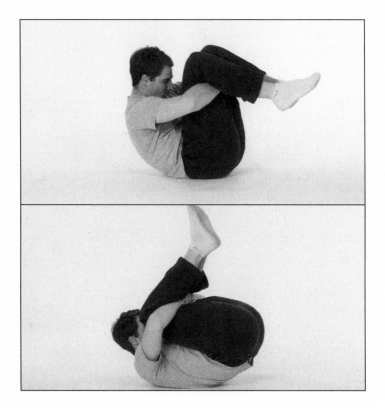

SET-UP

Tuck the knees into your chest and rock back and forth.

Wrist/Forearm Stretches
Feel it Here Wrist

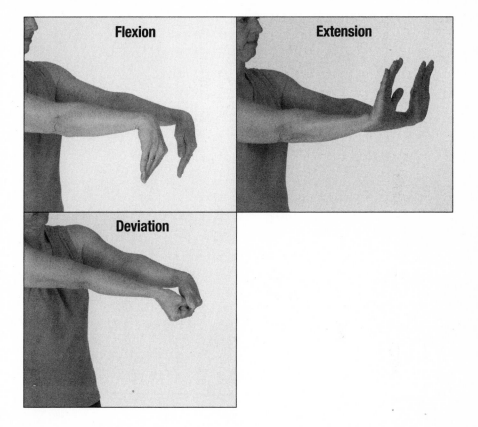

SET-UP

Flexion (Pullover): Gently provide traction to the wrist by pulling out on the hand. This will create the sensation of your hand and forearm moving away from one another. Assist the movement from the back of the middle part of the hand.

Extension (Pullback): Gently pull out on the wrist. Draw back the fingers and hand together. To intensify the stretch, pull back closer to the fingers.

Deviation (Thumb Pull): Begin by tucking the thumb into the palm of the hand. Cup the fingers of the stretching wrist around the thumb. Assist the wrist in tilting downwards while keeping the elbow straight.

Lateral Neck Stretch

Feel it Here Neck, Shoulder

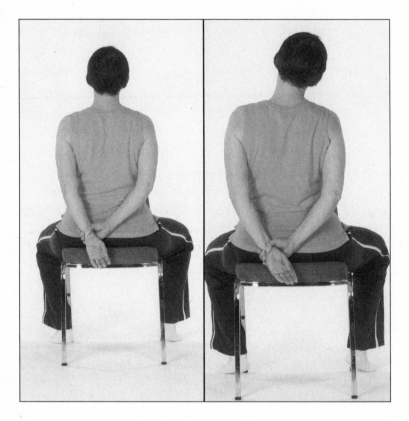

SET-UP

Sit with the arm of the shoulder to be stretched placed behind you. Gently drop your ear to your other shoulder. Then, grab the wrist of the shoulder/ neck area being stretched. Relax the opposite side shoulder by breathing deeply into the side being stretched. Allow your head to return to neutral before releasing the wrist.

Double Arm Torso Stretch

Feel it Here Middle Back, Hips, Shoulders

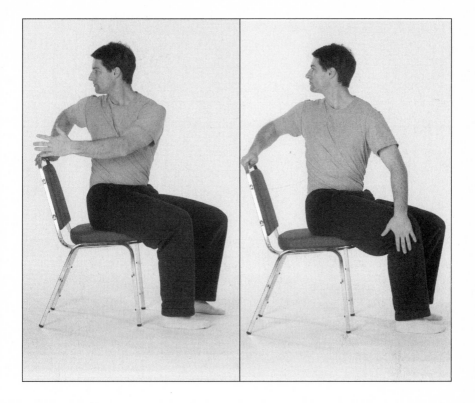

SET-UP

Begin with your hands on the top of a chair back positioned at shoulder height. Slide your hands a bit wider than the shoulders. Staying loose through the middle back and hips, hinge at your hips and drop your chest forward through the arms. If you feel pinching or tightness around the neck or shoulders rotate your palms so they are facing palms in.

Counter Rotation with Bent Knee

Feel it Here Middle & Lower Back, Hips, Chest/Shoulder Area

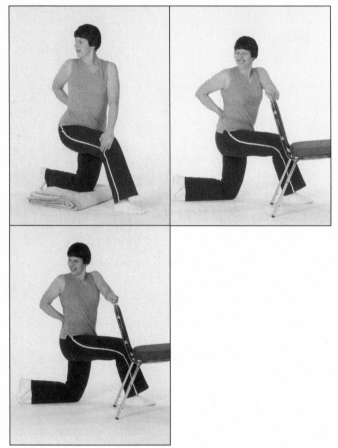

SET-UP
Find an elevated surface such as a step or bench. Place your foot on the surface keeping your ankle, knee, and hip aligned. Stand as upright as possible emphasizing rotation through your middle back, not the lower back. Place your hand across your knee to assist in rotation. If you have difficulty rotating across your body, you can perform this exercise against a chair, as shown above.

Doggy Door

Feel it Here Groin, Hips

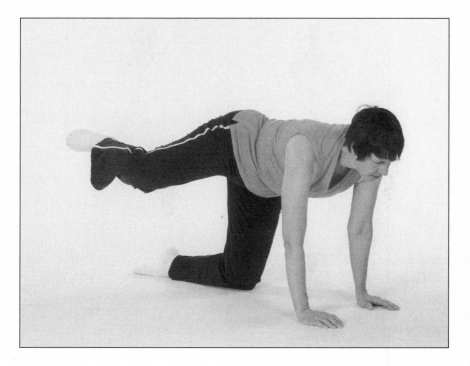

SET-UP

Keep you core active to stabilize your back and hips. Keeping the non-lifting hip firm into the ground, lift the opposite knee with the outside hip muscle. Be careful not to shift your weight to the non-working side.

Double Arm Hug Rotation

Feel it Here Upper & Middle Back

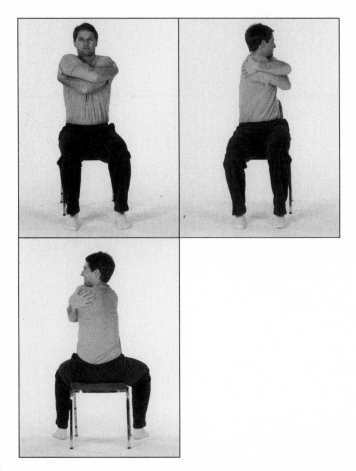

SET-UP

Sit upright on a sturdy surface. Give yourself a 'big hug'. Keeping pressure on the backs of the shoulders, rotate around your waist.

Alphabet Series: L's

Feel it Here Shoulders, Middle Back

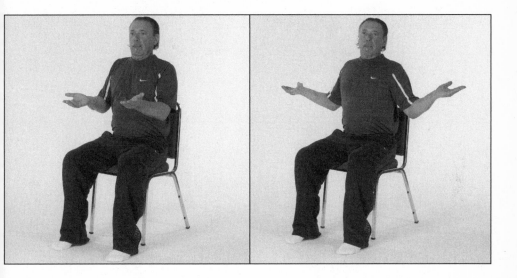

SET-UP

Sit upright on a sturdy surface. Squeeze your shoulder blades back and down. Maintain this position while rotating the shoulders and keeping your hands out and together.

Alphabet Series: W's

Feel it Here Middle Back

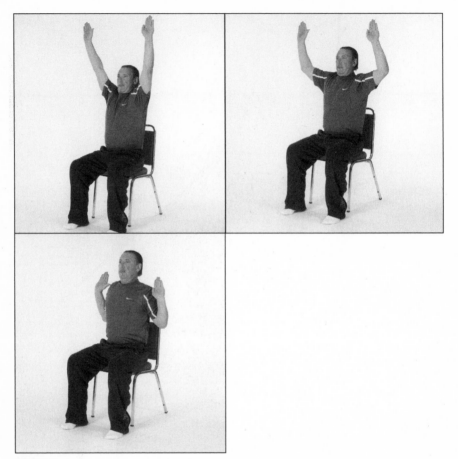

SET-UP

Sit upright on a sturdy surface. Squeeze your shoulder blades back and down. Draw both elbows down and back into the middle spine. Hold, then release.

Alphabet Series: Y's

Feel it Here Middle & Lower Back

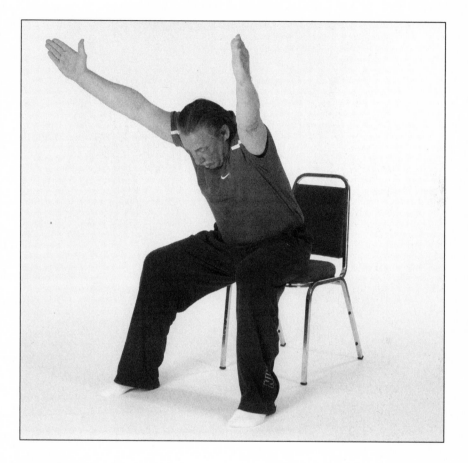

SET-UP

Sit upright on a sturdy surface. Squeeze your shoulder blades back and down. Draw both arms up, and straight out in front of your body at a 45 degree angle.

Alphabet Series: T's

Feel it Here Middle Back, Behind Shoulders

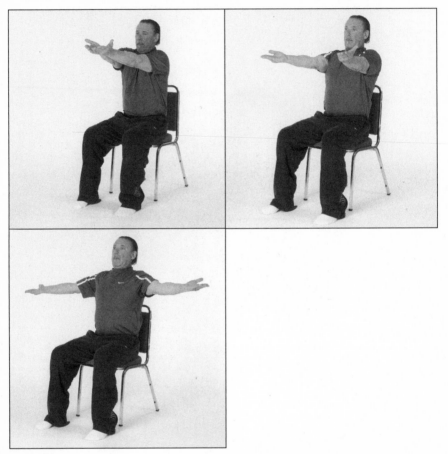

SET-UP
Sit upright on a sturdy surface. Squeeze your shoulder blades back and down. Draw both arms out from the mid-line of the body with palms up.

Glutes

Feel it Here Outer Hip, Lower Back, Hamstrings

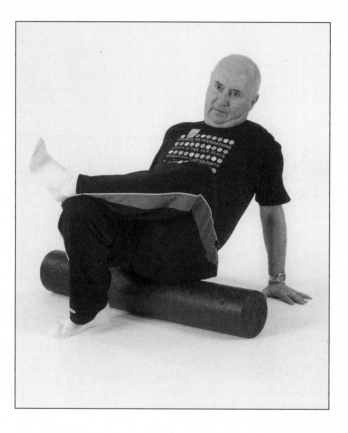

SET-UP

Position your outer hip on the roller. Apply pressure into the roller with the hip, and slowly rotate the hip from the knee.

Rotator Cuff Stretch

Feel it Here Shoulders

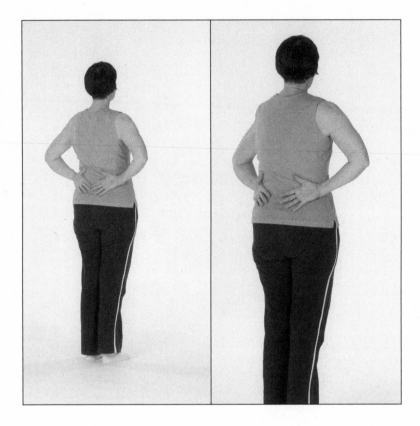

SET-UP

Shake out the shoulders. Gently press the outside of your hands into the lower back, while allowing the elbows to drift forward. Upon reaching an end point, return the elbows back to neutral and slide the hands down and out.

Ribcage Opener

Feel it Here Groin, Back, Shoulders

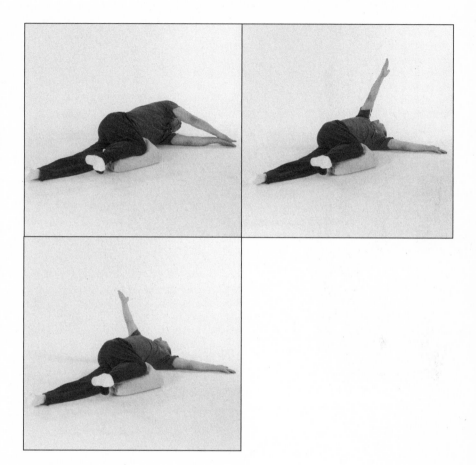

SET-UP
Lay on the ground and position a rolled up towel or foam roller under your knee. Start with your hands together. Press your knees into the object then initiate rotation with your hand. Follow the rotation down the arm until you feel it through your ribcage.

Prone Extension Lifts

Feel it Here Middle of Back, Lower Back, Hips

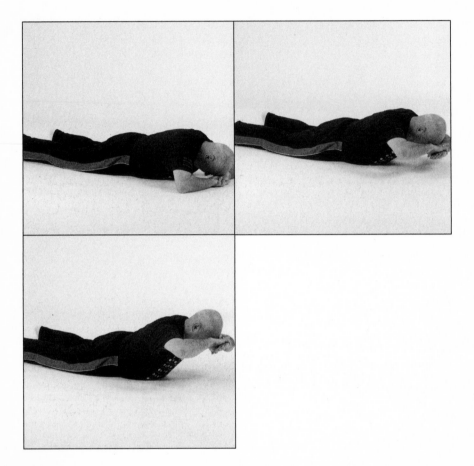

SET-UP
Lay face down, positioning your hands, palms down, against your forehead. Keep your head in light contact with your hands and lift from your middle back one vertebrae at a time.

Cranial Release

Feel it Here Neck

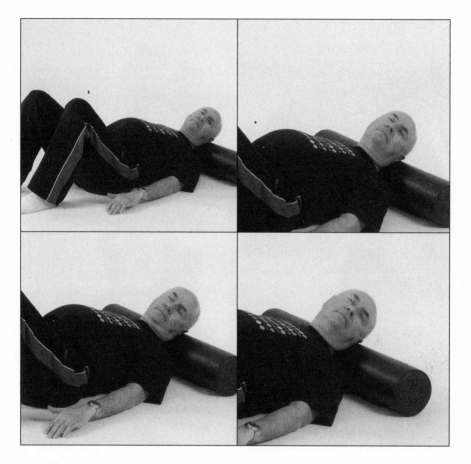

SET-UP

Lay on your back. Position the back of your head, right where it meets the base of your neck, on the roller. You should be in a comfortable position; draw your feet into your hips if needed. Your hands should be relaxed near the sides of your hips. If you need to stabilize the roller, place your hands on the sides of the roller. Rotate your head to the right and left. When rotating your head to the right and left, feel the small space that sits on either side of your head. Keep pressure in the roller by slightly extending your neck, emphasizing proper alignment. *Check out www.meltmethod.com*

Sacral Release

Feel it Here Pelvis

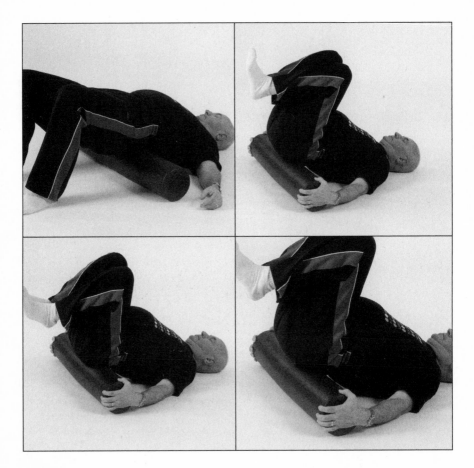

SET-UP

Position your body in a comfortable bridging position on your spine. Elevate your hips and slide the roller on your sacrum. Keeping your ribs heavy (see page 56), engaging your core, pull one knee at a time up to a position over your hips. Addressing one side of your pelvis at a time, let your knees drift over until you feel a 'barrier' or place of irritability. Once found, gently make circles with your knees both ways, then switch to the other side. *Check out www.meltmethod.com*

Foam Roller Scissor Stretch

Feel it Here Core, Lower Back

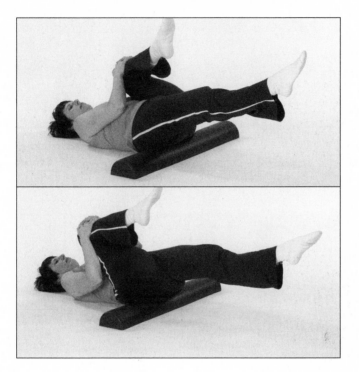

SET-UP

Lay on your back with your knees bent and feet close to your hips. Press your feet into the floor, then elevate your hips. Slide a foam roller (or very thick towel) beneath your tailbone/sacrum. Keeping your ribs heavy (see page 56), pull one knee to your chest and hold. Extend the leg next, keeping ribs heavy, engaging the core. The sacrum is the flattish bone that positions itself directly below the lower back. Place the palm of your hand on the sacrum; it should fit nicely. The roller sits between the lower back and sacrum. *Check out www.meltmethod.com*

Adductors with Roller

Feel it Here Inner Thigh

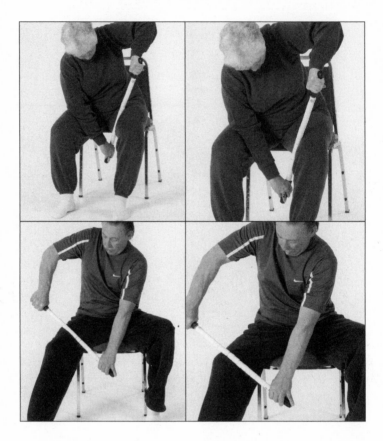

SET-UP

Position your upper inner thigh on the roller. Applying pressure into the roller with the leg, flex and extend the knee. Proceed to move down the roller to the next "barrier" and repeat the same flex/extend movement.

Calf Raises

Feel it Here Calves, Feet

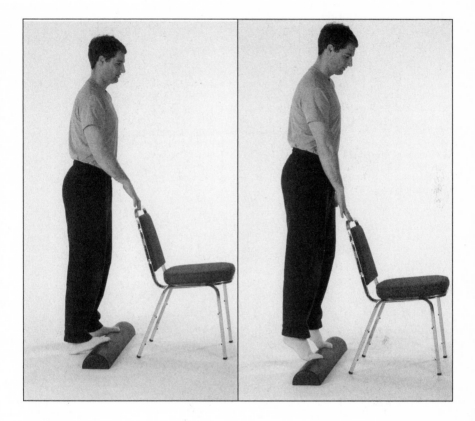

SET-UP

Stand atop a foam roller, facing a chair with your feet parallel and pointed forward. You should be able to see the front of your feet when looking down. Keep your hands light against the chair. Begin by pressing the balls of your feet into the ground, then pull your heels up towards the back of your hips. To increase the effort on the calves and feet, perform the movement higher off the ground and on a single leg.

87

Physio-ball Foot Lifts

Feel it Here Hips, Legs

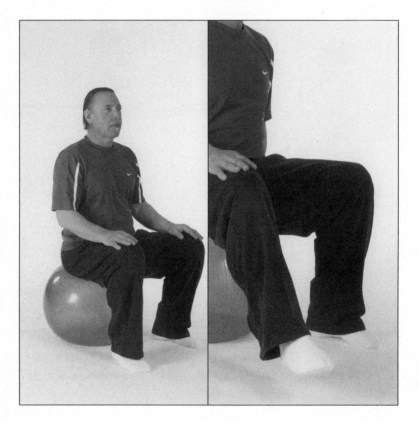

SET-UP

Sit on the very top of the Physio-ball. You should feel as if you are sitting slightly higher than on a regular chair and a bit more open in the front of the hips. Use the hip hinging cue (see page 57) to find the back alignment necessary to maintain positioning and stability. Feel braced through the core. This will stabilize your back and hips before you lift your foot. Lift one foot off the floor, hold. Work on shifting your body weight slowly to one foot prior to lifting the opposing knee/foot. Use a mirror or partner to accomplish.

Lateral Ball Roll

Feel it Here Glutes, Legs, Spine

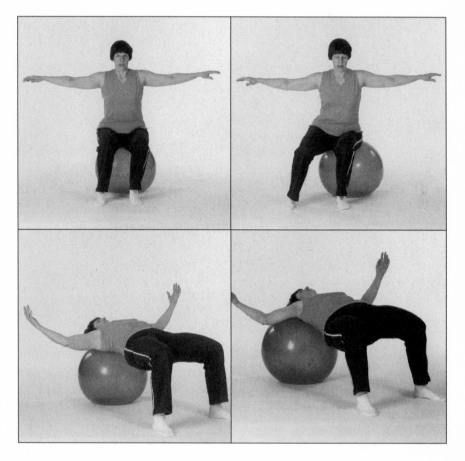

SET-UP

Begin sitting upright on the Physio-ball. Keep your feet in front of your hips and "walk" to the left on the ball. Repeat to the right side. The on-back version will be completed in the same manner, but your beginning position will be on your back.

89

Physio-ball Rotational Twists

Feel it Here Spine, Back

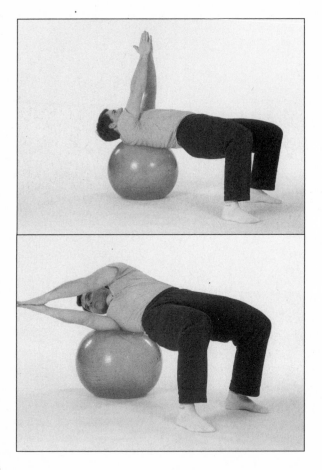

SET-UP

Sit on the highest point of the Physio-ball. Keeping your feet steady, walk down until your shoulders and head are resting comfortably on the ball. You will be positioned in a bridge position with emphasis placed on the hips, feet, and back muscles for stability. Keep the hips up by imagining you're squeezing a piece of paper between your glutes, which flattens out the hips. Don't let your hips drop! Press your hands together and initiate the twisting movement from your shoulders and core until your shoulders are stacked. Stacking the shoulders will indicate you've reached your end point.

90

Physio-ball Walk-up

Feel it Here Legs, Hips, Core

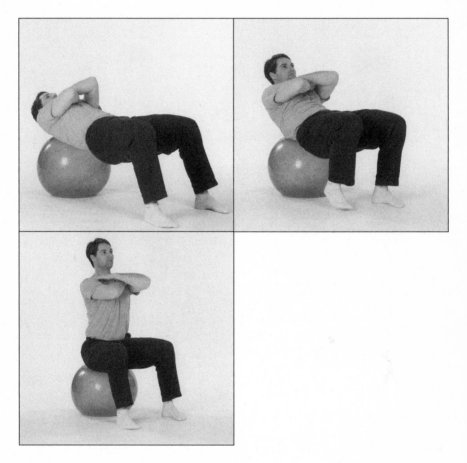

SET-UP

Position your hips on top of the Physio-ball. Brace your core. Walk up the ball using your full foot. Keeping the feet wider adds stability if you feel off balance during the up or down phases.

Open Hip Squats

Feel it Here Groin, Hips, Legs, Lower Back

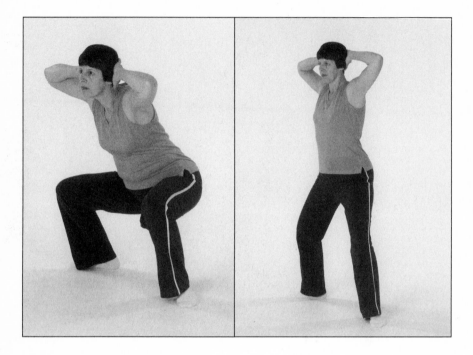

SET-UP

Start in a standard squatting position with your toes positioned at 11 and 1 o'clock. Keeping your back straight, initiate the opening of the hips from the legs. Drop the hips down and back into the squat.

Kegel

Feel it Here Pelvic Floor, Core

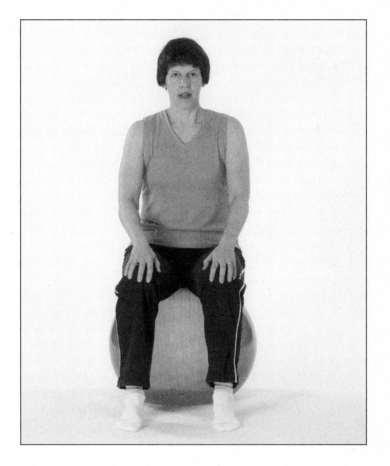

SET-UP

While keeping your lower back quiet and relaxed, squeeze your pelvic floor muscles in and up towards the pelvis. Imagine there is a balloon attached to your pelvic floor and its rising. Try this exercise on the floor first to take surrounding muscles out of the learning curve.

93

All Fours Core Progression

Feel it Here Core, Middle/Lower Back

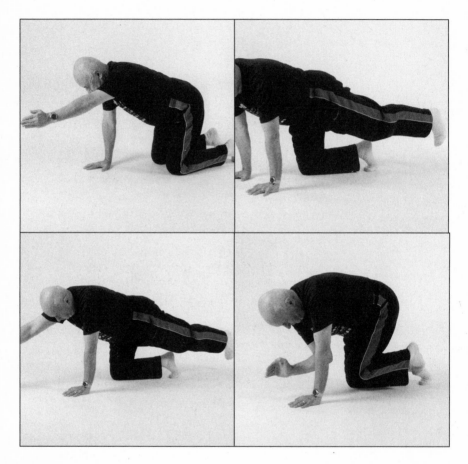

SET-UP

Begin the core series on all fours. Each progression will begin with ribs heavy (see page 56) and bracing the core as you draw your navel to your spine. To draw the navel in, imagine squeezing a marble in your belly button. Use a rolled up towel to keep your core active during the progressions. A small Physio-ball can be placed under your spine if you feel your back muscles are tightening up. This variation helps your body isolate movements and learn faster.

Forward Plank

Feel it Here Stomach, Legs, Shoulders

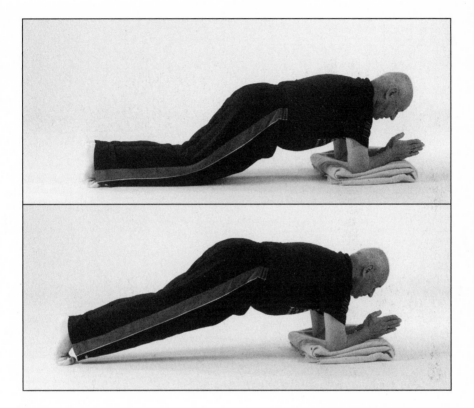

SET-UP

Position your body in the same position as a push-up, but with your hands positioned together in front of your face. To help cue the pulling of the navel to the spine, place a rolled up towel on your lower back as a bio-feedback tool. Make sure you are breathing through the entire movement. Pull your navel to the lower spine but do not flatten your lower back out. Instead, cue the lower ribs to become 'heavy'.

95

Spiderman

Feel it Here Groin, Hips, Core, Spine

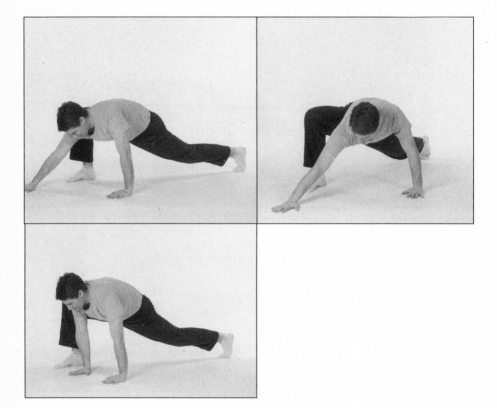

SET-UP

Begin in the push-up position. Gently bring one foot forward to stretch the opposite sides of the body, keeping your chest upright and spine long through the motion. Alternate this movement by stepping forward and backward.

Chopping Movements

Feel it Here Core, Hips

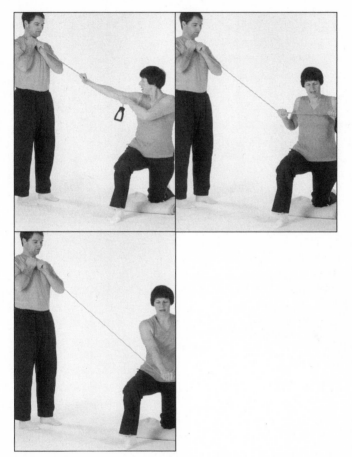

SET-UP

Chop across your body over a trailing, kneeling leg. Your front knee is on the ground on a towel or other comfortable item. Pull the band into your body, then push it down and out with the trail hand. Keep your spine neutral by concentrating on bracing your stomach and stabilizing the hips. Think about moving around a stable pillar in your spine.

Exercise provided by St. John's, AAHFRP, FMS

97

Lifting Movements

Feel it Here Core, Hips

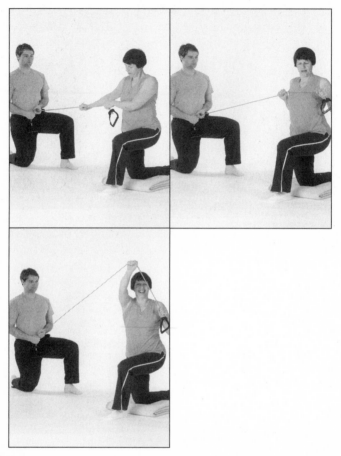

SET-UP

You will be lifting across your body over a trailing knee on the ground. The front knee should be aligned with your hip. Pull the band into your body, then push it up and out with the trailing hand. Keep your spine neutral by concentrating on bracing your stomach and stabilizing the hips. Think about moving around a stable pillar in your spine.

Exercise provided by St. John's, AAHFRP, FMS

Draw the Sword /Return the Sword

Feel it Here Back of Shoulder, Middle Back

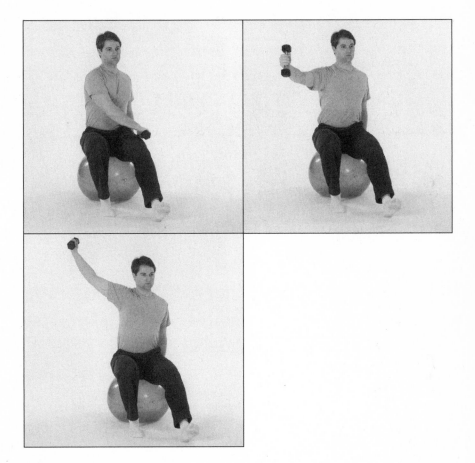

SET-UP

Imagine you are drawing a sword from the opposite side with a closed hand. Draw the sword across your body into an open hand position over the opposite shoulder. The motion is accomplished with the back muscles. The muscles run from the back of the shoulder through the middle back. Imagine your shoulder has a direct line of action drawn from the shoulder to the opposite hip. For an alternative, hold a light weight (shown above) in the hand that moves across the body.

Band Pulls

Feel it Here Arms, Back, Core

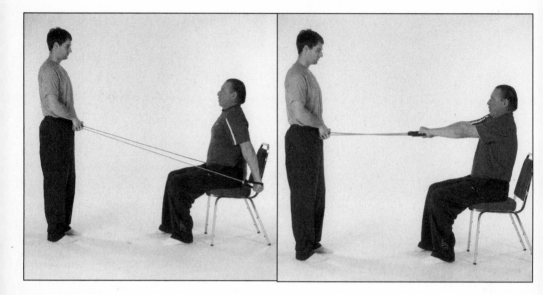

SET-UP

Keep the weight of your body in the feet and hips by slightly leaning forward. This allows the shoulders and arms to move naturally. Cue the shoulder blades to stay back and down thereby relaxing the upper neck muscles.

Inch Worm Walk-up

Feel it Here Shoulders, Core, Legs

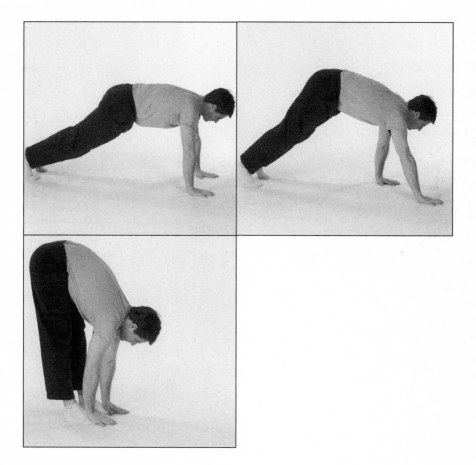

SET-UP

Beginning in a pike position, walk your hands forward until you reach the starting position for a push-up. Brace your stomach then walk your hands back toward the feet. Do not allow your back to sag once the push-up position is reached. Keeping your hands moving together during this movement is important.

Band Rows

Feel it Here Back, Shoulders, Core

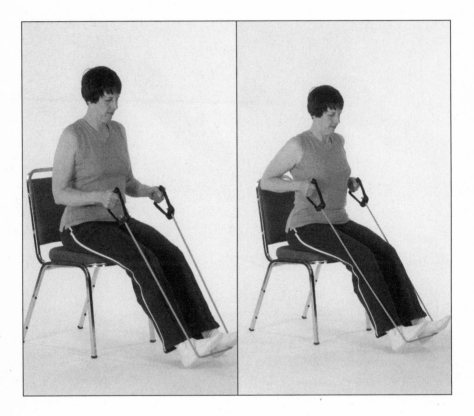

SET-UP

Position your body in an upright position on either a ball or bench. First, pull your shoulder blades back. Keeping them back, pull one elbow back at a time. Keep your ribs heavy (see page 56) and core contracted during each pressing repetition. Breathe out during each rep and breathe in upon return to the starting position. This exercise can also be done while standing.

Front Pullbacks

Feel it Here Core, Arms, Chest, Legs

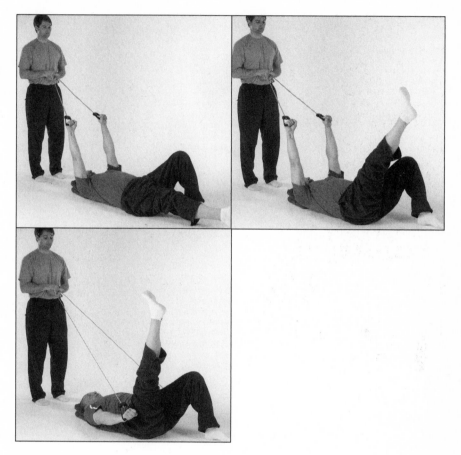

SET-UP

Begin this exercise on your back. Keeping your ribs heavy, initiate this movement from your core. Pull both arms toward one leg, pause, and return. Brace prior to each repetition.

Stability Hold in Push-up

Feel it Here Core, Shoulders, Legs

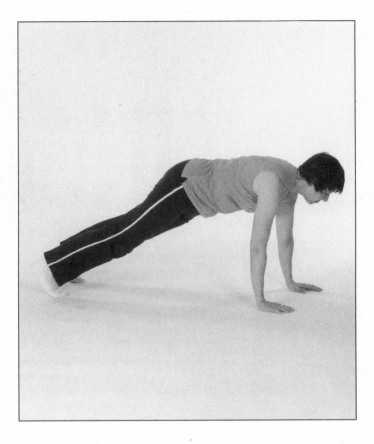

SET-UP

Assume a push-up position. Brace your core, be strong through your spine, and balanced on your hands and feet.

Band Pulls Across Body

Feel it Here Back, Shoulders, Core

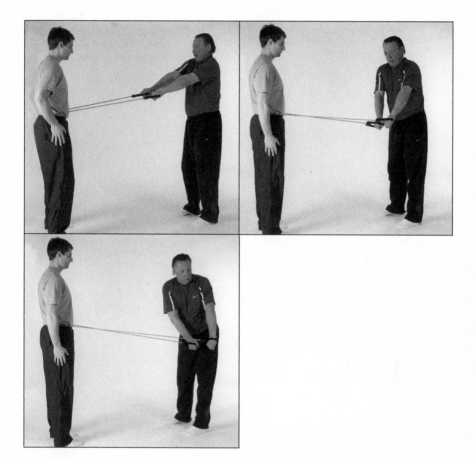

SET-UP

Assume a neutral hip stance. Keep equal weight distribution on both legs throughout the exercise. Pull both hands across the body staying in a somewhat upright position.

Double Arm Chest Press

Feel it Here Chest, Shoulders, Arms

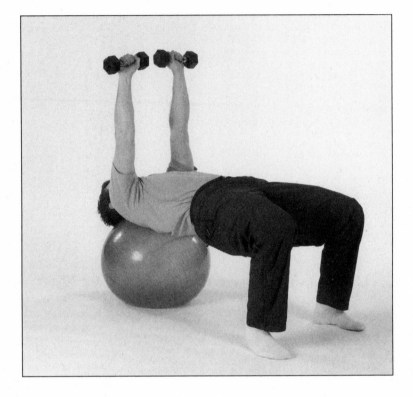

SET-UP

Lay on your back. Start the set with the dumbbells extended in front of you. Bring both down toward the outside of your shoulders. Pause, and return the dumbbells to the starting position. For a variation of this movement try sitting on a Physio-ball to start. You will feel your back and hips working more during this movement.

Curling and Pressing Combo

Feel it Here Arms, Shoulders

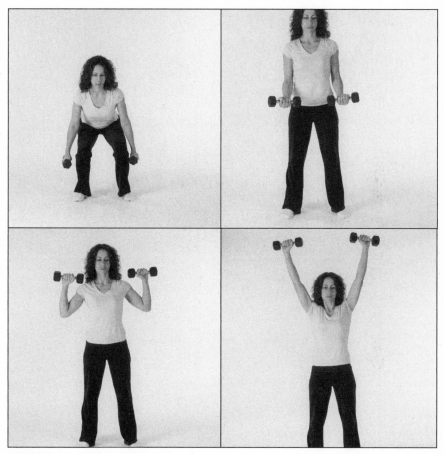

SET-UP

Position yourself in a half-squat position. Dumbbells should be by the sides of your body. Brace your core. Curl the dumbbells up first and then, press them above your head, keeping your shoulders in a neutral position.

Row with Tricep Extension

Feel it Here Back, Triceps

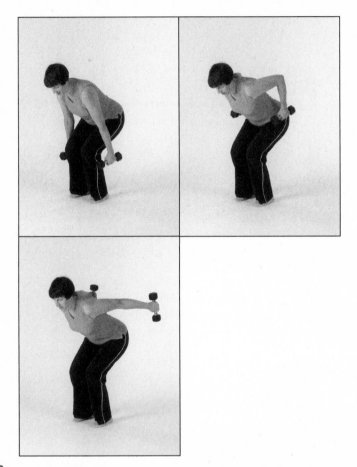

SET-UP

Either kneel (and use one arm) or stand and use both arms, shown above.
Perform a row, pulling your elbows behind your back and then extend your
arm fully in back of you to work the triceps.

Lateral Lunge with Shoulder Press

Feel it Here Hips, Knees, Ankles

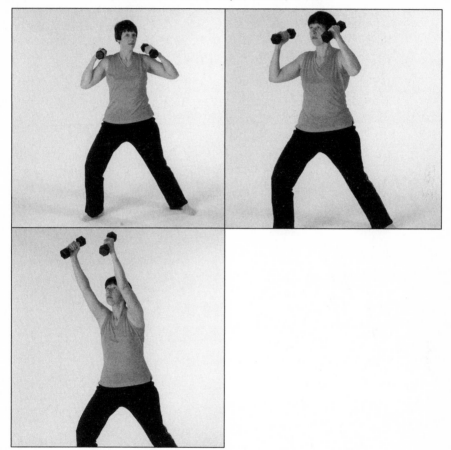

SET-UP

Lunge to the side, sitting back into the exercise. Upon returning to the starting position, press the dumbbells across the body. Be sure to keep your back straight and your shoulders squared forward.

Deadlift

Feel it Here Hips, Legs, Back

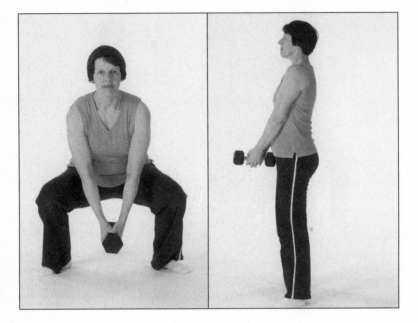

SET-UP

Squat with a dumbbell between your legs and perform the deadlift, slowly lifting the dumbbell up as you straighten your legs.

Single Leg Deadlift

Feel it Here Glutes, Hamstrings

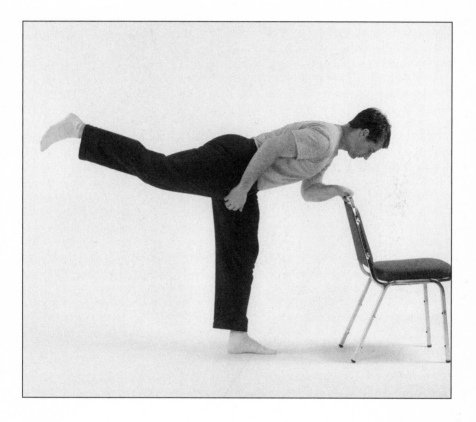

SET-UP

Draw one leg back straight while keeping your hips square. Perform the deadlift while keeping the leg off the floor. Use a wall or chair for assistance in balancing.

Chest Stretch Open Arms

Feel it Here Chest, Shoulders

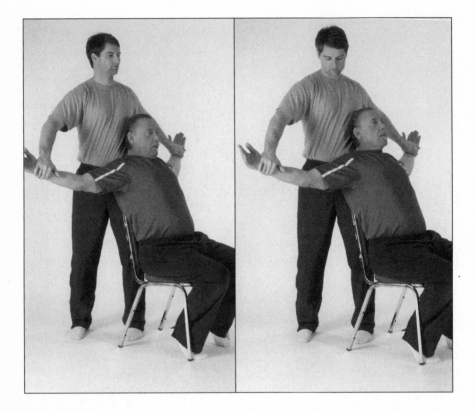

SET-UP
Stand behind your partner with your hands gently placed upon his or her upper arms. Keep your body positioned along your partner's spine to stabilize and assist in creating a greater stretch through the front of your partner's body.

Shoulders/Torso Stretch

Feel it Here Chest, Core, Shoulders

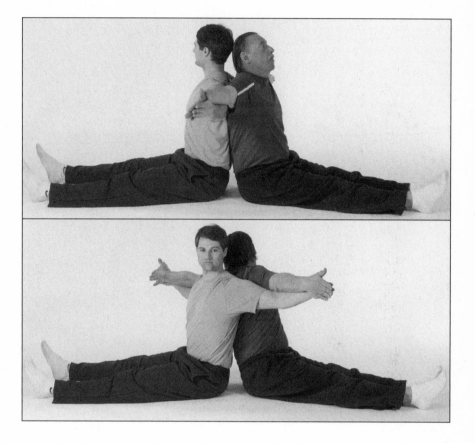

SET-UP

Sit back to back with your partner. Place palms in contact and rotate in unison.

Back to Back Butterfly Stretch

Feel it Here Groin, Hips

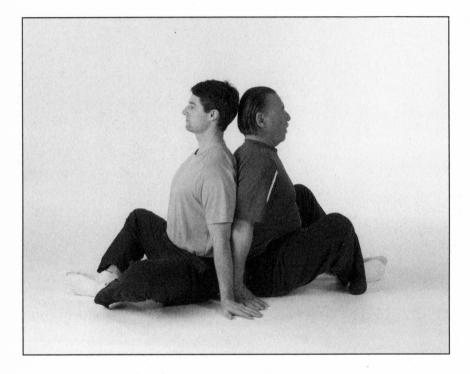

SET-UP

Sit back to back with your partner in the butterfly position, with your legs out to the side to stretch your inner thighs and hips.

Assisted Rotational Lunge Stretch

Feel it Here Hips, Torso

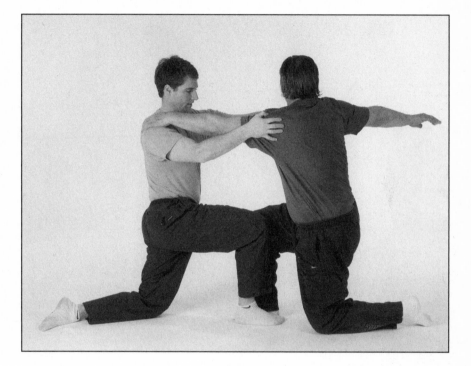

SET-UP
Facing your partner, lunge forward and make contact with your inner thighs. Upon feeling pressure in the groin, assist your partner's rotation across the knee.

Double Hand Chest Press

Feel it Here Chest, Arms, Core

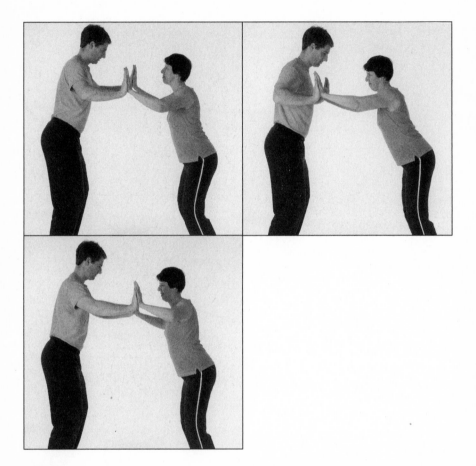

SET-UP

Press your palms against your partner's. Press your hands back and forth, resisting one another, but still allowing for range of motion similar to a dumbbell chest press. Be sure to stabilize backward through your core.

116

Single Hand Chest Press

Feel it Here Chest, Shoulders, Arms

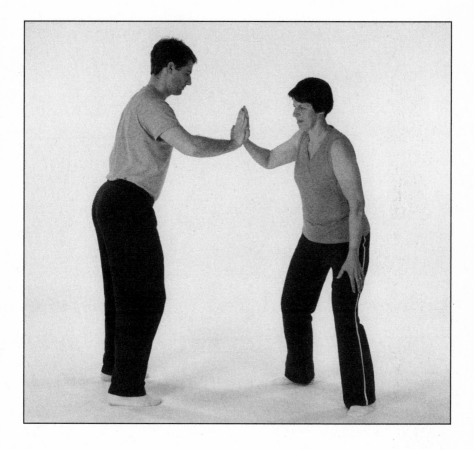

SET-UP

Using only one arm, press the palms of your hands against your partner's. Press the hands back and forth, resisting one another, but still allowing for range of motion similar to a dumbbell chest press. Be careful not to over push your partner's arm too hard and be sure to stabilize forward and backward through your core.

Partner Abduction

Feel it Here Outside Hip, Lower Back

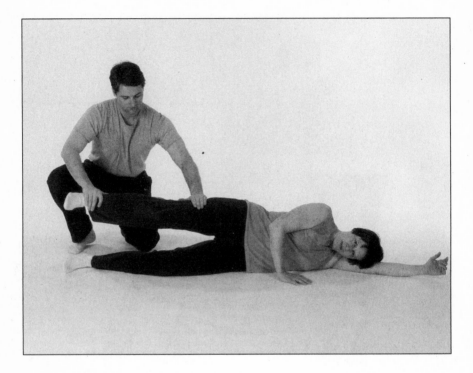

SET-UP

Push your leg up, while your partner applies pressure against the outside of the ankle. Be sure to cue your partner to keep the quad snug to stabilize the knee.

118

Partner Adduction

Feel it Here Inside Groin, Hips

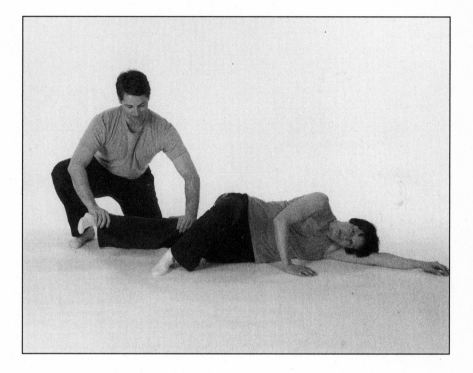

SET-UP
Apply pressure against the inside of your partner's leg as the leg is being pulled across the midline of the body. Be sure to cue your partner to keep the quad snug to stabilize the knee.

119

CHAPTER SEVEN

Exercise Programs and Progressions

Warm-up/Warm-down refers to the number of minutes that should be taken to warm-up your body before a set of exercises and then the time to warm-down your body. For example, 4/4 means you take 4 minutes to warm-up and 4 minutes to warm-down.

Rest refers to the time taken between each set of exercises.
RPE refers to Rate of perceived Exertion. See page 37 for details.

Preparatory Phase Program

Length: 2 Weeks x 6 Routines
Exercise Time:

Weeks 1-2   30 minutes/session
Weeks 3-4   40 minutes/session

Complete the exercises in each category top to bottom, with 2 sets of 10 reps each. Frequently re-visit the exercises you enjoy, too!

RPE: 5/10
Tempo (seconds): 2 up/2 down

Week 1

Category	Exercise	Page #	Equipment
Stability	Deep Breathing Technique*		
Stability	Kegel	93	Physio-ball
Stability	Lateral Plank	53	
Movement	Physio-ball Roll	61	Physio-ball
Movement	Counter Rotation with Bent Knee	72	Chair (optional)
Stamina	Walk for 15-20 minutes		

*Deep Breathing Technique: Breathe into your collarbones, back, pelvic floor, and ribs.

Week 2

Category	Exercise	Page #	Equipment
Stability	Deep Breathing Technique (see page 122)		
Stability	Hip Hinging	57	Physio-ball
Stability	Forward Plank	95	
Movement	Alphabet Series	75-78	Chair
Movement	Double Arm Torso Stretch	71	Chair
Stamina	Walk for 20-25 minutes		

Beginner Level I Program

Length: 1-4 weeks
Total Weekly Activity Time: 4 Hours Max
Exercise Time: 2 Hours (Structured)
Leisure Time: 2 Hours (Unstructured)
Be sure to complete each exercise and category completely with 1-2 sets of 8 reps each.
RPE: 5-6
Warm-up/Warm-down: 4/3
Rest: 2 min.

Category	Exercise	Page #	Equipment
Movement	Standing Tail Wag	50	
Movement	Spinal Whip	58	
Balance	Calf Raises	87	Chair
Balance	Physio-ball Foot Lifts	88	Physio-ball
	Push-up	52	Dowel (optional)
	Chair Sit	51	Chair
	Standard Lunge	60	
	Band Pulls Across Body	105	Theraband
	Band Pulls	100	Theraband
	Walk for 2 minutes (heart rate down to 10 beats for resting heart rate)		
Flexibility	Double Arm Hug Rotation	74	Chair
Flexibility	Assisted Rotational Lunge Stretch	115	

Beginner Level II Program

Length: 5-8 weeks
Total Weekly Activity Time: 4 Hours Max
Exercise Time: 2 Hours (Structured)
Leisure Time: 2 Hours (Unstructured)

Be sure to complete each exercise and category completely with 2 sets of 10 reps each.

RPE: 5-6
Warm-up/Warm-down: 3/3
Work/Rest: 1/2

Category	Exercise	Page #	Equipment
Core	Deep Breathing Technique (see page 122)		
Mobility	Ribcage Opener	81	
Mobility	Alphabet Series	75-78	Chair
Movement	Prone Extension Lifts	82	
Movement	Physio-ball Walk-ups	91	Physio-ball
	Push-up	52	Dowel (optional)
	Walking for 2 minutes (heart rate down to 10 beats for resting heart rate)		
Flexibility	Lateral Neck Stretch	70	Chair

Intermediate Level I Program

Length: 5-8 weeks
Total Weekly Activity Time: 4 Hours Max
Exercise Time: 2 Hours (Structured)
Leisure Time: 2 Hours (Unstructured)

Be sure to complete each exercise and category completely with 2 sets of 12 reps each.

RPE: 6-10
Warm-up/Warm-down: 10/5
Work/Rest: 1/2

Category	Exercise	Page #	Equipment
Mobility	Hip Hinging	57	Physio-ball
Mobility	Spinal Whip	58	
Movement	Lateral Ball Roll	89	Physio-ball
Strength	Double Arm Chest Press	106	Dumbbells
Strength	Curling and Pressing Combo	107	Dumbbells
	Lateral Plank	53	
	Wrist/Forearm Series	69	
	Cranial Release	83	Foam roller
	Thoracic Flex on Roller	62	Foam roller
	Walk for 3-4 minutes (if time allows)		

Note: Revisit Kegels (page 93) or Deep Breathing (page 122) throughout your workout progressions.

Intermediate Level II Program

Length: 9-12 weeks
Total Weekly Activity Time: 4.5 Hours Max
Exercise Time: 2.5 Hours (Structured)
Leisure Time: 2 Hours (Unstructured)

Be sure to complete each exercise and category completely with 2-3 sets of 10 reps each.

RPE: 6-10
Warm-up/Warm-down: 8-10/5
Work/Rest: 1/1.5

Category	Exercise	Page #	Equipment
Mobility	Alphabet Series	75-78	
Mobility	Open Hip Squats	92	
Movement	Physio-ball Rotational Twists	90	Physio-ball
Strength	Band Pulls Across Body	105	Theraband
Stability	Chopping Movements	97	Theraband
Stability	Lifting Movements	98	Thereband
Movement	Sacral Release	84	Foam roller
Movement	Adductors with Roller	86	Roller
	Deep Breathing (see page 122)		

Note: Revisit Childs Pose (page 59), Tail Wag (page 50) and Draw the Sword (page 99) during your workout progressions.

Advanced Level I Program

Length: 13-16 weeks
Total Weekly Activity Time: 5 Hours Max
Exercise Time: 2.5 Hours (Structured)
Leisure Time: 2.5 Hours (Unstructured)

Be sure to complete each exercise and category completely with 2-3 sets of 12 reps each.

RPE: 7
Warm-up/Warm-down: 8/5
Work/Rest: 1/1

Category	Exercise	Page #	Equipment
Movements	Spinal Whip	58	
Movements	Physio-ball Rotational Twists	90	Physio-ball
Movements	Spiderman	96	
Stability	Deadlift	110	Dumbbell
Stability	Row with Tricep Extension	108	Theraband
Stability	Push-up (2 sets only)	52	Dowel (optional)
Warm-down	Bent Knee Hamstring	63	Theraband
Warm-down	Adductors with Band	64	Theraband

Note: Revisit Thoracic Flex (page 62), foam rolling series (pages 79, 83-84, 86) and balance exercises (pages 87-91) throughout your workout progressions.

Advanced Level II Program

Length: 17-20 weeks
Total Weekly Activity Time: 5 Hours Max
Exercise Time: 2 Hours (Structured)
Leisure Time: 3 Hours (Unstructured)

Be sure to complete each exercise and category completely with 3 sets of 10 reps each.

RPE: 7-8
Warm-up/Warm-down: 8/5
Work/Rest: 1/1

Category	Exercise	Page #	Equipment
Movements	Childs Pose	59	
Stability	All Fours Core Progression	94	
Movements	Roll and Hold	68	
Stability	Lateral Lunge w/ Rotational Shoulder Press	109	Dumbbells
Stability	Physio-ball Walk-ups	91	Physio-ball
Stability	Push-up (2 sets only)	52	Dowel (optional)
Warm-down	Foam Rolling series (1 min per) (add scissor stretch #)	79, 83-84, 86	Foam Roller
Warm-down	Deep Breathing (see page 122) or Walk for 2 minutes		

Note: Revisit Spidermans (page 96), Foam Rolling series (pages 79, 83-84, 86) and balance exercise section (pages 87-91) throughout your workout progressions.

Stamina

Beginner Level I

Length: 1-4 weeks
Total Weekly Activity Time: 2 Hours Max

Be sure to complete each exercise and category completely with 1 set of 8 reps each.

RPE: 5-6
Warm-up/Warm-down: 4/4

Category	Exercise	Page #	Equipment
Mobility	Overhead Squat	44	Dowel, Foam Roller
Cardiovascular Health	15 minutes of bike riding, vigorous walking, aquatics, or dancing		
Core	All Fours Core Progression	94	
Core	Lateral Plank	53	
Hips	Doggy Door	73	
Hips	Standing Tail Wag	50	

Strength Circuit

Beginner Segment

Reps: 8
Sets: 1
RPE: 5-6

Category	Exercise	Page #	Equipment
Beginner Strength 1	Prone Extension Lifts	82	
Beginner Strength 1	Lateral Plank	53	
Beginner Strength 1	Forward Plank	95	
Beginner Strength 2	Stability Hold in Push-up	104	
Beginner Strength 2	Chair Sit	51	Chair
Beginner Strength 2	Band Rows: Sitting	102	Theraband, chair

Intermediate Segment

Reps: 10
Sets: 2
RPE: 6

Category	Exercise	Page #	Equipment
Intermediate Strength 1	Draw the Sword/ Return the Sword	99	Physio-ball, light weight
Intermediate Strength 2	Inch Worm Walk-ups	101	
Intermediate Strength 2	Band Rows: Standing	102	Theraband

Advanced Segment

Reps: 10
Sets: 3
RPE: 7

Category	Exercise	Page #	Equipment
Advanced Strength 1	Band Pulls	100	Theraband
Advanced Strength 1	Band Pulls Across Body	105	Therband
Advanced Strength 2	Chopping Movements	97	Theraband
Advanced Strength 2	Lifting Movements	98	Theraband

Posture Circuit
Beginner Segment

Reps: 8
Sets: 1
RPE: 6

Category	Exercise	Page #	Equipment
Beginner Posture 1	Standard Lunge	60	
Beginner Posture 1	Ribs Heavy	56	Foam Roller
Beginner Posture 1	Lifting Technique	98	Small weight
Beginner Posture 2	Alphabet Series: L's	75	Chair
Beginner Posture 2	Rolling Technique from Floor	55	

Intermediate Segment

Reps: 10
Sets: 2
RPE: 6

Category	Exercise	Page #	Equipment
Intermediate Posture 1	Thoracic Flex on Roller	62	Foam Roller
Intermediate Posture 1	Childs Pose	59	
Intermediate Posture 2	Double Arm Chest Press	106	Dumbbells
Intermediate Posture 2	Prone Extension Lifts	82	

Advanced Segment

Reps: 12
Sets: 2
RPE: 7

Category	Exercise	Page #	Equipment
Advanced Posture 1	Physio-ball Rotational Twists	90	Physio-ball

Shoulder Girdle Circuit

To do a complete circuit workout, do an entire segment of exercises. For example, a Beginner's Shoulder Girdle Circuit would include all the exercises listed below for Beginner Shoulders 1. The WU/WD is 4/4 and the W/R is 1/2 for these circuits.

Beginner Segment

Reps: 8
Sets: 1
RPE: 5-6

Category	Exercise	Page #	Equipment
Beginner Shoulders 1	Spinal Whip	58	
Beginner Shoulders 1	Childs Pose	59	
Beginner Shoulders 1	Ribcage Opener	81	

Intermediate Segment

Reps: 10
Sets: 2
RPE: 6

Category	Exercise	Page #	Equipment
Intermediate Shoulders 1	Alphabet Series: L's	75	Chair
Intermediate Shoulders 1	Rotator Cuff Stretch	80	
Intermediate Shoulders 1	Ribcage Opener	81	

Advanced Segment

Reps: 12
Sets: 2-3
RPE: 6

Category	Exercise	Page #	Equipment
Advanced Shoulders 1	Front Pullbacks	103	Theraband
Advanced Shoulders 1	Stability Hold in Push-up	104	
Advanced Shoulders 1	Draw the Sword /Return the Sword	99	Physio-ball, light weight

Balance Circuit

Beginner Segment

Reps: 8
Sets: 1
RPE: 5-6

Intermediate Segment

Reps: 10
Sets: 2
RPE: 6

Category	Exercise	Page #	Equipment
Beginner Segment	Calf Raises	87	Chair
Beginner Segment	Lateral Ball Roll	89	Physio-ball
Beginner Segment	Physio-ball Walk-ups	91	Physio-ball
Intermediate Segment	Heel to Toe Walking	49	
Intermediate Segment	Lateral Ball Roll	89	Physio-ball

Hip Circuit

To do a complete circuit workout, do an entire segment of exercises. For example, a Beginner's Hip Circuit would include all the exercises listed below for Beginner Hips 1 and 2. The WU/WD is 4/4 and the W/R is 1/2 for these circuits.

Beginner Segment

Reps:　8
Sets:　1
RPE:　5

Category	Exercise	Page #	Equipment
Beginner Hips 1	Standing Tail Wag	50	
Beginner Hips 1	Back to Back Butterfly Stretch	114	
Beginner Hips 1	Bent Knee Hamstring	63	Theraband
Beginner Hips 2	Adductors with Band	64	Theraband
Beginner Hips 2	Chair Sit	51	
Beginner Hips 2	Hip Lifters	66	

Intermediate Segment

Reps:　10
Sets:　2
RPE:　6

Category	Exercise	Page #	Equipment
Intermediate Hips 1	Abductors	65	Theraband
Intermediate Hips 1	Chair Sit	51	
Intermediate Hips 1	Glutes	79	Foam Roller
Intermediate Hips 2	Windshield Washer	67	Towel
Intermediate Hips 2	Foam Roller Scissor Stretch	85	Foam Roller

Advanced Segment

Reps: 15
Sets: 2
RPE: 7

Category	Exercise	Page #	Equipment
Advanced Hips 1	Sacral Release	84	Foam Roller
Advanced Hips 1	Lateral Ball Roll	89	Physio-ball
Advanced Hips 2	Adductors with Band	64	Theraband
Advanced Hips 2	Bent Knee Hamstring	63	Theraband
Advanced Hips 2	Roll and Hold	68	

Partner Workout Circuit

Workout   Maintenance

	Workout	Maintenance
Reps:	10	12
Sets:	2	2-3
RPE:	6	6-7

Category	Exercise	Page #	Equipment
Stretching*	Chest Stretch Open Arms	112	Chair
Stretching*	Shoulders/Torso Stretch	113	
Stretching*	Back to Back Butterfly Stretch	114	
Stretching*	Assisted Rotational Lunge Stretch	115	
Strength	Double Hand Chest Press	116	
Strength	Single Hand Chest Press	117	
Strength	Partner Abduction	118	
Strength	Partner Adduction	119	

*Hold stretching exercises for 10-12 seconds.

Assessments

INITIAL EVALUATION DATE (WEEK 1):
MID-POINT EVALUATION DATE (WEEK 4):
SUMMARY EVALUATION DATE (WEEK 9):

Functional Evaluation

	ABLE TO COMPLETE?	DISCOMFORT FELT?	NOTE DIFFICULTY
	YES/NO	YES/NO	YES/NO
Overhead Squat			
Getting up from Chair (no hands)			
Stair Walking (optional no hands)			
Standing Eyes Open/ Closed (2-legs)			
Getting up from Ground			
Heel to Toe Walking			

Physical Evaluation

	GOAL	INITIAL	MID-POINT	SUMMARY
Chair Sit.	1 Minute			
Push-ups	20 Max			
Forward Plank	45 Secs			
Lateral Plank	45 Secs			
Quarter Mile Timed Walking	2 Mins 30 Secs			
12 minute Walking Test	1.25 Miles			

Appendix

Stress Screening

The Miller & Smith Stress Test

A number of years back, Miller and Smith developed a simple test that helps determine if stress is currently playing a role in your life and, if not, whether you are prone to developing stress-related health complications down the line.

Directions: Score each item from 1 (always) to 5 (never), according to how much of the time each statement applies to you.

1 (Always) **2** (Almost Always) **3**(Periodically) **4** (Almost Never) **5** (Never)

1. ___ I eat at least one hot, balanced meal a day.
2. ___ I get 7 to 8 hours of sleep at least four nights a week.
3. ___ I give and receive affection regularly.
4. ___ I have at least one relative within 50 miles.
5. ___ I exercise to the point of perspiration at least twice a week.
6. ___ I smoke less than half a pack of cigarettes a day.
7. ___ I take fewer than 5 alcoholic drinks a week.
8. ___ I am the appropriate weight for my height.
9. ___ I have an income adequate to meet basic expenses.
10. __ I get strength from my religious beliefs.
11. __ I regularly attend club or social activities.
12. __ I have a network of friends and acquaintances.
13. __ I have one or more friends to confide in about personal matters.
14. __ I am in good health (including eyesight, hearing, and teeth).
15. __ I am able to speak openly about my feelings when angry or worried.
16. __ I have regular conversations with the people I live with about domestic problems, chores, money, daily living issues.
17. __ I do something for fun at least once a week.
18. __ I am able to organize my day effectively.
19. __ I drink fewer than three cups of coffee (or tea, or cola drinks) a day.
20. __ I take quiet time for myself during the day.
_____ TOTAL RAW SCORE

TOTAL RAW SCORE - 20 =_____ VULNERABILITY SCORE

SCORING: To get your score, add up all of the numbers and subtract 20. Any number over 30 indicates a vulnerability to stress. You are seriously vulnerable if your score is between 50-75, and extremely vulnerable if it is over 75.

Health Chart

Name William Smith	Sleep	Resting Heart Rate	Blood Pressure	Waist Circum	BMI	Cholesterol
Date:			AM: PM:			

To determine your BMI (Body Mass Index), use the formula below:

$$BMI = \frac{weight\ (lb)\ x\ 702}{height^2\ (in^2)}$$

After you have found your BMI, use that measurement to find where your BMI lies on the chart below.

BMI	
18.4 or less	Underweight
18.5 – 24.9	Normal
25 – 29.9	Overweight
30 or greater	Obese

For example, a 5'4" woman weighing 135 pounds would have a BMI of:

BMI = (135 x 703) / (64)
     = 23.17

According to the chart above, this woman's BMI of 23 falls within the normal range.

Recommended Nutritional Intake

The table below provides recommendations for your daily intake of each nutrient, based on a 2000 calorie diet.

NUTRIENT	UNIT OF MEASURE	DAILY VALUES
Total Fat	grams (g)	65
Saturated fatty acids	grams (g)	20
Cholesterol	milligrams (mg)	300
Sodium	milligrams (mg)	2400
Potassium	milligrams (mg)	3500
Total carbohydrate	grams (g)	300
Fiber	grams (g)	25
Protein	grams (g)	50
Vitamin A	International Unit (IU)	5000
Vitamin C	milligrams (mg)	60
Calcium	milligrams (mg)	1000
Iron	milligrams (mg)	18
Vitamin D	International Unit (IU)	400
Vitamin E	International Unit (IU)	30
Vitamin K	micrograms (µg)	80
Thiamin	milligrams (mg)	1.5
Riboflavin	milligrams (mg)	1.7
Niacin	milligrams (mg)	20
Vitamin B6	milligrams (mg)	2.0
Folate	micrograms (µg)	400
Vitamin B12	micrograms (µg)	6.0
Biotin	micrograms (µg)	300
Pantothenic acid	milligrams (mg)	10
Phosphorus	milligrams (mg)	1000
Iodine	micrograms (µg)	150
Magnesium	milligrams (mg)	400
Zinc	milligrams (mg)	15
Selenium	micrograms (µg)	70
Copper	milligrams (mg)	2.0
Manganese	milligrams (mg)	2.0
Chromium	micrograms (µg)	120
Molybdenum	micrograms (µg)	75
Chloride	milligrams (mg)	3400

Supermarket Checklist

Use the checklist below to help you stock your pantry and fridge with the most useful—and healthy—ingredients. This will make it even easier for you to create well-balanced meals for yourself and your family.

BEANS/LEGUMES
(low-sodium canned or dry)
- [ ] Hummus
- [ ] Black Beans
- [ ] Kidney Beans
- [ ] Garbanzo

CONDIMENTS
- [ ] Dijon Mustard
- [ ] Tamari
- [ ] Soy Sauce
- [ ] Ponzu Sauce
- [ ] Salsa
- [ ] Ketchup

DAIRY (organic)
- [ ] Organic butter
- [ ] Eggs, omega 3 enriched
- [ ] Skim Milk
- [ ] Cheese, low fat
- [ ] Yogurt

FRUITS and VEGETABLES
- [ ] Berries, fresh or frozen
- [ ] Dried Fruit of choice
- [ ] Fruit of choice, pineapple, peach or cantaloupe
- [ ] Lemon, lime (for juice and slices)
- [ ] Salad greens of choice
- [ ] Vegetables of choice (for sandwiches,

PROTEINS
- [ ] Chicken
- [ ] Beef Tenderloin
- [ ] Turkey
- [ ] Salmon

MISCELLANEOUS
- [ ] Coconut Milk
- [ ] All-Fruit Preserves
- [ ] Protein powder

NUTS/SEEDS
All natural butter
(almond, cashew, or peanut)
- [ ] Almonds
- [ ] Flax Seeds
- [ ] Walnuts
- [ ] Pumpkin Seeds

OILS and FATS
- [ ] Cold pressed extra virgin olive oil

SPICES and HERBS
- [ ] Brown Sugar
- [ ] Cinnamon Sticks
- [ ] Chili powder
- [ ] Garlic, fresh
- [ ] Ginger
- [ ] Rosemary
- [ ] Thyme
- [ ] Pepper
- [ ] Salt, sea
- [ ] Sugar

STOCKS
- [ ] Vegetable stock
- [ ] Chicken stock
- [ ] Beef stock
- [ ] Vegetable stock

SWEETENERS
- [ ] Honey
- [ ] Maple Syrup
- [ ] Blackstrap Molasses

VINEGARS
- [ ] Balsamic vinegar
- [ ] Rice Vinegar
- [ ] Apple Cider Vinegar

WHOLE GRAIN PRODUCTS
- [ ] Whole grain cereal of choice
- [ ] Brown Rice
- [ ] Couscous
- [ ] Whole Wheat Breadcrumbs
- [ ] Whole Wheat crackers
- [ ] Whole Wheat Tortilla
- [ ] Whole Wheat Pita
- [ ] Quinoa
- [ ] Steel-Cut Oatmeal
- [ ] Other whole wheat grains

For more information on shopping for a healthy diet, turn to *Navigating the Supermarket: A Nutritious Guide to Shopping Well* by William Smith and Christina Wellington *(visit www.lulu.com to order).*

Equipment

OPTP
www.optp.com

Allegro Medical
www.allegromedical.com

Perform better
www.performbetter.com

Reference/Resources

American Association of Cardiovascular and Pulmonary Rehabilitation
www.aacvpr.org

American College of Cardiology
www.acc.org

American College
of Sports Medicine
www.acsm.org

American Heart Association
Exercise and Cardiac
Rehabilitation, and Prevention
Committee
www.americanheart.org

Center for Disease Control
www.cdc.gov

Cleveland Clinic Miller Family
Heart & Vascular Institute
*www.clevelandclinic.org/
heartcenter/pub/guide/prevention/
exercise/chooserehab.htm*

Framingham Heart Study
www.framingham.com/heart/profile.htm

Human Anatomy Online
www.innerbody.com

My Pyramid (USDA)
www.mypyramid.gov

National Institute on Aging
www.nia.nih.gov/

Post Rehab Online
www.postrehab.com

Pri-Med Patient Education Center
www.patientedu.org

Robert Wood Johnson Medical
School Division of Cardiovascular
Diseases and Hypertension
*www.rwjms.umdnj.edu/medicine/
cdh/clinical_programs.htm*

Texas Heart Institute
www.texasheartinstitute.org

World Health Organization
www.who.int/en/

GLOSSARY

Atherosclerosis
A disease where plaque forms on the insides of your arteries (National Heart Lung and Blood Institute).

Atria
The heart's upper chambers

Balance
A state of bodily equilibrium. Examples of activities that require balance are walking, getting up from a chair, and completing exercises. Coordination and balance tend to go hand in hand during movement.

Beta Blockers
Class of drugs that has various purposes, but particularly for the management of cardiac arrhythmias.

Blood Pressure
The pressure blood puts on the arteries. Produced mainly by the heart's contractions, blood pressure is measured with two numbers. Systolic pressure is taken after the heart contracts and is higher, while diastolic pressure is taken before the heart contracts..

Circulatory System
The system composed of the heart, arteries, capillaries, and veins that is responsible for moving oxygenated blood from the lungs and heart into the body through the arteries.

Cardio respiratory fitness (also called aerobic endurance or aerobic fitness)
The ability of the body's circulatory and respiratory systems to supply fuel and oxygen during sustained physical activity.

Chronic Disease
A disease that persists for a long time. According to the U.S. National Center for Health Statistics, a chronic disease must last 3 or more months.

Coronary Heart Disease
Also known as coronary artery disease, coronary heart disease occurs when the small blood vessels supplying blood and oxygen to the heart narrow. (National Library of Medicine)

Diuretic
Anything that promotes the formation of urine by the kidneys.

Exercise
A physical activity that is planned or structured. It involves repetitive bodily movement done to improve or maintain one or more of the components of physical fitness --cardio respiratory endurance (aerobic fitness), muscular strength, muscular endurance, flexibility, and body composition.

Heart
A hollow muscular organ that pumps blood through the body using rhythmic contractions.

Leisure-time physical activity
Exercise, sports, recreation, or hobbies that aren't associated with activities as part of one's regular job duties, household, or transportation.

Light-Intensity Activities
Activities performed with limited energy expenditure. Examples include walking slowly, swimming (slow treading), gardening, and bicycling (very light).

GLOSSARY

Metabolic Syndrome
Occurs when symptoms appear at the same time, increasing the development of coronary artery disease, stroke, and Type 2 Diabetes.

Mobility
This term relates to both joint/s and global movement capacity. Each joint is meant to have proper mobility through its range of motion, whereby humans must have effective mobility to walk, run, and perform activities of daily living. Mobility becomes a major problem as we age.

Moderate-intensity physical activity
A level of effort in which a person should experience some increase in breathing or heart rate. Examples include walking briskly, golfing (pulling/carrying clubs), mowing lawn, recreational swimming, and resistance training exercise circuit.

Muscular Endurance
The capability the muscles have to continually perform without tiring. To improve your muscle endurance, try cardio respiratory activities such as walking, jogging, bicycling, or dancing.

Muscular Strength
The amount of force a muscle applies during an activity . The key to making your muscles stronger is working them against resistance, whether that is from weights or gravity.

Physical activity
Any bodily movement produced by skeletal muscles that result in an expenditure of energy.

Resting Heart Rate
This is a person's heart rate at rest. The best time to find out your resting heart rate is in the morning, after a good night's sleep, and before you get out of bed. At rest, your heart will beat about 60 to 80 times a minute (American Heart Association).

Risk Factors
Can be divided into negotiable (can be changed) and non-negotiable (can't be changed). Negotiable factors include smoking, cholesterol, blood pressure, and waist circumference. Non-negotiable include family history, age, and gender.

Stability
The quality, state, or degree of being stable.

Stamina
Resistance to fatigue, illness, hardship, etc.; endurance

Statins
A class of drugs that alter cholesterol levels in the blood.

Ventricles
The two chambers of the heart involved in pumping blood. The right ventricle pumps blood into the lungs to receive oxygen. The left ventricle pumps blood into the body's circulatory system, delivering oxygen to organs and tissues. (Medical Dictionary Online)

ABOUT THE AUTHORS

William Smith, MS, NSCA, CSCS, MEPD, completed his B.S. in exercise science at Western Michigan University followed by a master's degree in education and a post-graduate program at Rutgers University. In 1993 Will began coaching triathletes and working with athletes and post-rehab clientele. He was a Division I Collegiate Strength Coach and has been competing in triathlons and marathons since 1998, recently finishing the Steelhead Half Ironman in Michigan in 5 hours and 22 minutes. Will founded Will Power and Fitness Associates and currently consults for fitness, healthcare, and wellness centers in New York and New Jersey. The Director of the Professional Development Institute, Will has co-authored a book on triathalon training (*Tri-Power,* 2007) and his book *Exercises for Back Pain* will also be published later this year.

Dr. Fred M. Aueron is Board-Certified in Internal Medicine, Cardiovascular Diseases, and Interventional Cardiology. He is the New Jersey Governor of the Society of Cardiac Angiography and Interventions, a Fellow in the Society of Cardiac Angiography and Interventions and the American College of Cardiology.